Introduction to Phenomenology

To my mother, Nancy Tatano, who at 102 years of age is still an inspiration to me.

Introduction to Phenomenology
Focus on Methodology

Cheryl Tatano Beck
University of Connecticut

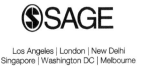

Los Angeles | London | New Delhi
Singapore | Washington DC | Melbourne

FOR INFORMATION:

SAGE Publications, Inc.
2455 Teller Road
Thousand Oaks, California 91320
E-mail: order@sagepub.com

SAGE Publications Ltd.
1 Oliver's Yard
55 City Road
London, EC1Y 1SP
United Kingdom

SAGE Publications India Pvt. Ltd.
B 1/I 1 Mohan Cooperative Industrial Area
Mathura Road, New Delhi 110 044
India

SAGE Publications Asia-Pacific Pte. Ltd.
18 Cross Street #10-10/11/12
China Square Central
Singapore 048423

Library of Congress Cataloging-in-Publication Data

Names: Beck, Cheryl Tatano, author.

Title: Introduction to phenomenology : focus on methodology / Cheryl Tatano Beck.

Description: Los Angeles : SAGE, [2021] Summary: "Phenomenology is a challenging method for many students to understand and apply. Introduction to Phenomenology: Focus on Methodology breaks down the history, methodology, and application so students can more easily write proposals and conduct phenomenological research. Author Cheryl Tatano Beck draws on her depth of experience in applying and teaching phenomenological methods to distill the method into a single guidebook for students and new researchers alike. This introductory book provides a clearer picture of phenomenology as method and its applications to social, behavioral, and health sciences, covering both interpretive and descriptive phenomenology from research design through analysis"—Provided by publisher.

Identifiers: LCCN 2019029854 | ISBN 9781544319551 (paperback) | ISBN 9781544319537 (epub) | ISBN 9781544319544 (epub) | ISBN 9781544319568 (ebook)

Subjects: LCSH: Phenomenology—Research—Methodology. | Qualitative research—Methodology.

Classification: LCC B829.5 .B338 2021 | DDC 142/.78—dc23

LC record available at https://lccn.loc.gov/2019029854

Acquisitions Editor: Leah Fargotstein
Editorial Assistant: Claire Laminen
Production Editor: Jyothi Sriram and Astha Jaiswal
Copy Editor: Beth Ginter
Typesetter: Hurix Digital
Proofreader: Caryne Brown
Indexer: Amy Murphy
Cover Designer: Candice Harman
Marketing Manager: Shari Countryman

20 21 22 23 24 10 9 8 7 6 5 4 3 2 1

Contents

Detailed Contents

List of Tables and Figures

Tables

Figures

Acknowledgments

I would like to sincerely thank the reviewers of this textbook for the care they took and the time they invested in reviewing both drafts. Their insightful comments certainly helped to strengthen this textbook. The publication of this book could not have been possible without the tremendous help I have received from the following editorial and production staff at SAGE who I want to especially thank:

Acquisitions Editor: Leah Fargotstein

Editorial Assistant: Claire Laminen

Content Development Editor: Chelsea Neve

Production Editor: Jyothi Sriram and Astha Jaiswal

Copy Editor: Beth Ginter

Typesetter: Hurix Digital

Proofreader: Caryne Brown

Indexer: Amy Murphy

Cover Designer: Candice Harman

Marketing Manager: Shari Countryman

Reviewers to Acknowledge

- Dr. Tyrone Bynoe, University of Michigan - Flint

- Davin J. Carr-Chellman, University of Idaho

- Suzanne S. Dickerson, Professor, University at Buffalo School of Nursing

- Luis Gomez, Fielding Graduate University

- Alexander Jun, Ph.D. Azusa Pacific University

- Basia Kielczynska, DMH, MSAc, MS, Tri-State College of Acupuncture

- Jason Lawson, University of Mary

- Kevin Partridge, Carleton University
- Lynde Paule, Walden University
- Katarzyna Peoples, Walden University
- Heidi M. Rose, Villanova University
- Tova Sanders, Northeastern University
- Vikash Singh, Montclair State University
- Paul Tremblay, Western University (Canada)
- Roxanne Vandermause, University of Missouri-St. Louis
- Bruce E. Winston, PhD, Regent University

About the Author

CHERYL TATANO BECK, DNSc, CNM, FAAN

Dr. Beck is a Distinguished Professor at the University of Connecticut, School of Nursing. She also has a joint appointment in the Department of Obstetrics and Gynecology at the School of Medicine. She received her Master's degree in maternal-newborn nursing and her certificate in nurse-midwifery from Yale University. Her Doctor of Nursing Science degree is from Boston University. She is a fellow in the American Academy of Nursing and is inducted into the Sigma Theta Tau International Nurse Researcher Hall of Fame. Over the past 35 years, Cheryl has focused her research efforts on developing a research program on postpartum mood and anxiety disorders. Postpartum depression and posttraumatic stress disorder due to traumatic childbirth have been the two arms of her research program. Based on the findings from her series of qualitative studies, Cheryl developed the Postpartum Depression Screening Scale (PDSS). She is a prolific writer who has published more than 150 journal articles. She also has published multiple American Journal of Nursing Books of the Year such as *Nursing Research: Generating and Assessing Evidence for Nursing Practice* of which is a co-author with Dr. Denise Polit. Other books she has written include *Traumatic Childbirth, Postpartum Mood and Anxiety Disorders: A Clinician's Guide, Developing a Program of Research in Nursing, Secondary Qualitative Data Analysis for the Health Sciences, Writing in Nursing: A Brief Guide,* and *Routledge International Handbook of Qualitative Nursing Research.*

Sara Miller McCune founded SAGE Publishing in 1965 to support the dissemination of usable knowledge and educate a global community. SAGE publishes more than 1000 journals and over 800 new books each year, spanning a wide range of subject areas. Our growing selection of library products includes archives, data, case studies and video. SAGE remains majority owned by our founder and after her lifetime will become owned by a charitable trust that secures the company's continued independence.

Los Angeles | London | New Delhi | Singapore | Washington DC | Melbourne

Introduction

What a valuable gift phenomenology is for qualitative researchers. No matter what experience a researcher is investigating, phenomenology allows a privileged view of the meaning of that experience from the perspective of the participants. The readers of your study will be able to walk a mile in the shoes of the participants to learn firsthand what that experience is like. For example, what is it like for a pregnant to be repeatedly battered by her partner? What is it like for a person to have to sell the family business? What is it like for a man to be diagnosed with prostate cancer? What are the experiences of women executives after returning to work from childbirth in a technology-sector setting? Such valuable insights into these and so many other experiences can be gained through phenomenology. Use of phenomenology is not discipline limited. Any discipline, be it in the Health Sciences, Business, Education, Anthropology, etc., will benefit from this type of qualitative research.

You may ask, "Why use phenomenology as a research approach?" It is a source for questioning the meaning of life and how persons live it. This qualitative approach extends scientific knowledge by prying open what researchers would ordinarily not question. In phenomenology, researchers attempt to put aside their past experiences, biases, everyday understanding, and presuppositions about what they are studying in order to learn to see the phenomenon with fresh eyes without those blinders on. Phenomenological researchers try to eliminate their biases so that they won't taint their study outcomes. Objectivity is critical in phenomenological studies. In objectivity, researchers try to remain faithful and oriented to the phenomenon being studied while avoiding their unreflective presuppositions. The lived experience is sought, which is the experience a person lives through before we take on a reflective view of it (van Manen, 2014). Getting at essences and away from researchers' biases is key in this qualitative approach.

Phenomenology aims at gaining a deeper understanding of the meaning of experiences in everyday life. Phenomenology uses particular experiences to inductively describe the general or universal essence, namely the heart and soul of the phenomenon. In phenomenological analysis, these individual experiences of participants are stripped away of the particulars to describe the essence of the experience, that is, what makes an experience what it is, and without it, it is not that experience. Based on the findings of phenomenological studies, effective interventions can be designed to yield the greatest impact. To be able to achieve these lofty goals of phenomenology, there is one caveat: Qualitative researchers must pay meticulous attention to its methodology.

This book has been a desire of mine for more than 20 years since I started teaching PhD students qualitative research methodology courses at the University of Connecticut. What I wished for each semester as I was filling out my required textbook order form for my courses was a textbook that concentrated on the different methodologies of descriptive and interpretive phenomenology. As a result, I needed to piece together multiple readings for my students on different phenomenological methodologies. I hope with the publishing of my textbook, other faculty and students will reap its benefits.

Many books have been published on the philosophy of phenomenology but not on its methodology. Yes, the philosophy of phenomenology that underpins research is critical, but attention must also be paid to methodology. There are two types of phenomenology: descriptive and interpretive phenomenology. In descriptive phenomenology, the essence of an experience is described. Interpretive phenomenology is also called hermeneutic phenomenology. Hermeneutics is the science of interpretation. Interpretation is viewed as critical to understanding. In hermeneutic phenomenology, understanding is achieved through co-constructing the data with the research participants as understanding is achieved through a continual movement between the parts and the whole of the text of the participants' descriptions.

Method slurring is a pervasive problem in qualitative research. Phenomenology is not exempt from this problematic issue. Often I have read phenomenological studies, for instance, where the researcher has combined aspects of more than one methodology together. Picking and choosing parts of different phenomenological methodologies and combining them in one study definitely lessens its methodological rigor. One reason for reviewers' rejecting a manuscript for publication in a journal is method slurring. Also, grant reviewers with expertise in qualitative research may assign a grant poor scores because of method slurring.

In a cross-disciplinary review of phenomenological studies to prepare for writing this book, it became apparent that often the studies lacked methodological rigor. For instance, though the study was labeled by its author as being a phenomenological study, there was no specific methodology identified. Was it a descriptive phenomenological study or interpretive? Depending on which type, whose approach was used? Giorgi? van Manen? Colaizzi? These studies appeared to be more like generic qualitative research that does not follow a specific qualitative design. In other studies, even though researchers did identify which phenomenological approach they used, they did not stay true to that methodology. For instance, in Giorgi's approach, the researcher should not go back to the participants to validate the findings. However, some researchers did report they returned to the participants for member checking even though they stated they were using Giorgi's methodology. With this book, it is my hope that method slurring in phenomenological research will be decreased. Primary sources for each methodology are included in this book that should be used to guide researchers. So this is some of my rationale for designing this book to concentrate on methodology.

The audience for whom this book was written spans both faculty and graduate students. Professors who teach qualitative methodology courses, graduate students, junior faculty who are conducting a phenomenological study for the first time, and also senior faculty who haven't taken any qualitative methods courses are all appropriate audiences for this book. This book is also cross-disciplinary. It is written for faculty and students from all disciplines where qualitative research is conducted. Examples of these disciplines include Nursing, Business, Sociology, Social Work, Psychology, Nutritional Sciences, Sports Management, Physiotherapy, Occupational Therapy, Medicine, and Education. Faculty, students, and qualitative researchers from across the globe will benefit from this book, which has an international perspective. For each different descriptive and interpretive phenomenological methodology described in this book, there are international examples of research that used that specific approach.

This book is divided into four parts. Part I briefly provides a beginning understanding of the philosophical underpinnings of the methodologies of descriptive and interpretive (hermeneutic) phenomenology. Part II focuses on descriptive phenomenology. It consists of four chapters describing Colaizzi, Giorgi, van Kaam, Moustakas's modification, and Dahlberg, Dahlberg, and Nyström's approaches. Part III concentrates on interpretive phenomenology. This section comprises four chapters: one each for van Manen, Benner, Dahlberg et al., and Smith, Flowers, and Larkin's methodologies. Part IV addresses evaluating, writing, and teaching phenomenology. The final chapter provides an example of using phenomenology to develop a research program. The Glossary follows the last chapter and gives definitions of the key terms found in this book. In the appendices can be found two study activities for students, plus both a descriptive and an interpretive phenomenological proposal.

Chapter 2

To provide a little more in-depth description of what each chapter covers, we will start with Chapter 2. In order to provide a foundation for both descriptive and interpretive phenomenology, Chapter 2 briefly focuses on philosophy. As stated earlier, there are many books published on phenomenological philosophy for readers to consult, so here only a cursory discussion is provided. In Chapter 2, four philosophers are presented: Edmund Husserl, Martin Heidegger, Maurice Merleau-Ponty, and Hans-Georg Gadamer. Their philosophies provide the underpinnings for the different methodologies that follow in this book.

Chapter 3

In Chapter 3, the spotlight shines on Paul Colaizzi's methodology of descriptive phenomenology. Each step involved in conducting a study using his approach is described. An example of a study based on Colaizzi's methodology from my research program on postpartum depression is detailed as an illustration. The chapter ends with examples of studies from a variety of disciplines across the globe whose researchers employed Colaizzi's approach. The purpose of these published studies and those included in the other chapters of this book is to illustrate details of how in reality studies are carried out using the focused methodology of each chapter.

Chapter 4

In Chapter 4, Amedeo Giorgi's descriptive phenomenological methodology is explained. The steps making up his approach are each described, and his study on jealousy is used to concretely illustrate his steps. Swedish researchers' study on the experience of being an autonomous individual while dependent on advanced medical technology is recounted to provide an example of Giorgi's methodology. Other international examples of published studies employing his approach are included in the chapter.

Chapter 5

Adrian van Kaam's descriptive phenomenological methodology is the focus in Chapter 5. His 12-step approach is addressed and is supplemented by interdisciplinary examples of published studies to illustrate his methodology. Moustakas's modification of van Kaam's approach is frequently used by qualitative researchers, and so his modification is also included in this chapter.

Chapter 6

In Chapter 6 can be found Karin Dahlberg, Helena Dahlberg, and Maria Nyström's reflective lifeworld research methodology. Their approach begins with the art of "bridling", where researchers reflect on their experiences so they do not go unnoticed in the research process. Dahlberg and colleagues prefer the term "bridling" over "bracketing." Their methodology provides two types of analysis: one for a descriptive phenomenological study and one for an interpretive study. The focus of this chapter is on descriptive phenomenology using their reflective lifeworld approach. The chapter ends with a comparison of the five descriptive phenomenological methodologies of Colaizzi, Giorgi, van Kaam, Moustakas, and Dahlberg et al.

Chapter 7

Part III starts with Chapter 7, which centers on Max van Manen's interpretive phenomenological methodology. Addressed here are the six phases of his approach. In order to provide concrete examples of the application of his methodology, some international published studies from various disciplines are described.

Chapter 8

In Chapter 8, Patricia Benner's interpretive phenomenology is the focal point. Her methodology consists of multiple interrelated strategies, including thematic analysis, searching for paradigm cases, and analysis of exemplars. International examples of published studies from Iran and Switzerland that incorporated Benner's approach are included in this chapter to help illustrate her methodology.

Chapter 9

Jonathan Smith, Paul Flowers, and Michael Larkin's interpretive phenomenological analysis (IPA) is concentrated on in Chapter 9. Their method comprises six steps, which are explained. Illustrating their approach are studies from the United States (U.S.), United Kingdom (UK), Canada, Israel, and Ireland.

Chapter 10

The focal point in Chapter 10 is the second of Dahlberg et al.'s reflective lifeworld research, this time explaining their hermeneutic approach. A study conducted by Dahlberg and colleagues on inadequate care in emergency units is described to illustrate this approach. Additional examples of studies conducted by researchers in Sweden are included. This chapter concludes with a comparison of the four interpretive phenomenological methodologies addressed in Part III.

Chapter 11

Part IV begins with Chapter 11 where the target is evaluating the rigor of qualitative research. The debate over the terminology of trustworthiness versus reliability and validity is explored. Strategies for enhancing the quality of qualitative inquiry according to different phases of a research study are outlined. Criteria from two guides that specifically evaluate a phenomenological study are presented.

Chapter 12

Once a phenomenological study is complete, researchers' attention turns to the challenging task of writing. This is the focus of Chapter 12. There is an artistic craft involved in writing up phenomenological research in order to bring the riches of the findings to life. Creative strategies for presenting qualitative results are provided in this chapter along with specific examples of diagrams, figures, and tables I have used in publishing my own phenomenological studies.

Chapter 13

Chapter 13 addresses developing a program of research using phenomenology. The previous chapters in this book have focused on conducting a single phenomenological study. In this chapter, I wanted to provide an example of how researchers can develop a research program using a series of phenomenological studies they have systematically conducted. One option for using these studies is to develop a middle-range theory.

Chapter 14

As faculty, we have a responsibility to prepare the next generation of phenomenological scholars. Here faculty teaching strategies come into play. Chapter 14 is devoted to teaching phenomenology. Teaching approaches that have been published are described. Next I share examples of my own teaching assignments in my qualitative methodology courses that I use with my PhD students at the University of Connecticut.

GLOSSARY

Key terms used in phenomenological research are defined here for quick reference.

APPENDICES

In the appendices are two study activities for students. The first activity (Appendix A) directs students to choose one of the phenomenological methodologies described in this textbook and conduct an interdisciplinary search using various databases for phenomenological studies that used this approach. Students are then asked to select one study that is of interest to them and critique its methodology. Students can share their studies with the rest of the class. The second student activity (Appendix B) focuses on each student's discipline. Using the primary database for their discipline, such as ERIC for education, students report on the number of published phenomenological studies in their discipline. Which specific phenomenological approaches are used most often by qualitative researchers in their discipline? In appendices C and D can be found one example of a descriptive phenomenological proposal and one for an interpretive phenomenology proposal that can be used as examples for students.

REFERENCES

van Manen, M. (2014). *Phenomenology of practice*. Walnut Creek, CA: Left Coast Press, Inc.

PART I

Philosophical Underpinnings of the Methodology

Philosophy of Phenomenology

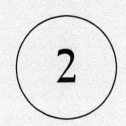

2

This chapter provides an introduction to the philosophy of phenomenology in order to provide the underpinnings for descriptive and interpretive (hermeneutic) phenomenological research methodologies. A discussion of the following prominent philosophers is included in this chapter: Edmund Husserl, Martin Heidegger, Maurice Merleau-Ponty, and Hans-Georg Gadamer.

....

EDMUND HUSSERL

Edmund Husserl is referred to as the father of the philosophy of phenomenology. He explained that his phenomenology was a descriptive philosophy of the essence of pure experiences. In *Cartesian Meditations* (1973a), Husserl declared that only knowledge that comes from immediate experiential evidence can be accepted. The crisis of science for Husserl (1970) was the loss of its meaning for life. "Scientific, objective truth is exclusively a matter of establishing what the world, the physical as well as the spiritual world, is in fact. But can the world, and human existence in it, truthfully have a meaning if the sciences recognize as true only what is objectively established in this fashion?" (pp. 6–7)

Husserl called for scientists to interrupt their natural attitude for a phenomenological attitude where the lifeworld is still present, but now we do not take it for granted; instead we question it. Natural attitude involves our taken-for-granted experiences as we live through them without reflective awareness. A new attitude was needed that was entirely different from the natural attitude in experiencing and thinking. Husserl (1983) called for a pure or transcendental phenomenology, which would not be a science of facts but instead, a science of essences, an eidetic science. Essence is what makes a phenomenon what it is, and without it, it would not be that phenomenon. Husserl called on the use of free imaginative variation to develop the discovery of the essence of an experience. In free imaginative variation, a person mentally removes an aspect of the phenomenon to determine if that removal transformed the phenomenon in an essential way. If it does, that aspect is considered essential, but if the phenomenon is still recognizable, it is not considered an essential part. One seeks the possible meanings of an experience through viewing it from divergent perspectives and different positions. The push here is to move away from just facts and let imagination help uncover meanings and essences. Husserl (1931) called this the play of fancy: "The pure essence can be exemplified intuitively in the data of experience, data of perception, memory, and so forth, but just as readily also in the mere data of fancy . . . intuitions rather of a merely imaginative order" (pp. 50–51).

To achieve this, one must go "back to the things themselves, to consult them in their self-givenness and to set aside all prejudices alien to them" (Husserl, 1983, p. 35). In the natural attitude, the world is continually there for us; it is "on hand." It is a naïve approach to viewing the world where persons take for granted the world as they perceive it. Here one views the world from a mainly uncritical position and does not consciously analyze what is experienced. In the natural attitude, persons evaluate their present experience in terms of their past experiences. Husserl claimed that instead of remaining in this natural attitude, we need to radically modify it. We need to put it out of action, put parentheses around the natural world that is on hand and continually there for us. Husserl termed this "the method of parenthesizing" or phenomenological reduction (Husserl, 1983, p. 60). Husserl admitted this requires a different turn. He claimed phenomenology was the first philosophy to require freedom from presuppositions and to call for a phenomenological attitude. One interrupts their natural attitude. The experiences of the world are still there, but now one critically reflects on his or her experiences and no longer takes them for granted.

The epoché and reduction are key elements in Husserl's philosophy of phenomenology. Epoché is the Greek word that means abstention. Husserl used this term to capture the actions required to suspend the natural attitude of taken-for-granted beliefs and the attitude of science. As a mathematician, Husserl borrowed the familiar word, bracketing, to more concretely provide the image of putting parentheses around our various presuppositions and assumptions that can hinder our being open to the meaning of phenomena. Bracketing is the means to achieving reduction, which comes from the word *re-ducere*, which means to lead back. The epoché opens up a different new kind of experience that Husserl (1973a) called a transcendental experience. Bracketing helps keep a tension between a researcher's past and present. It helps prevent researchers from being distracted by their presuppositions.

Phenomenological reduction for Husserl (1981) reveals a sweeping, unsuspected field of research. He went on to explain that if reduction is missing, lost is the opportunity to enter into a new realm. Husserl claimed that when one suspends the naïve exploration of the world, it doesn't mean you turn your back on the world to "retreat into an unworldly, and, therefore, uninteresting special field of theoretical study. On the contrary, this alone enables you to explore the world radically and even to undertake a radically scientific exploration of what exists absolutely and in an ultimate sense." (p. 322)

Husserl's (1970) transcendental epoché was meant to be a habitual attitude and not a temporary one. He emphasized that we must constantly deny ourselves our natural attitude. It is only through the epoché that the gaze of the philosopher is fully free.

Another main theme of Husserl's phenomenology was intentionality, which refers to the relationship between an individual and the object of his/her experience. It is a person's directed awareness of an object or event. For Husserl, intentionality means that our consciousness is oriented externally to the things of the world. Consciousness is not anything by itself, but instead consciousness is always being conscious of something. In intentionality, we direct our awareness to an object or event, to the experience of the world. Intentionality includes experiential horizons that Husserl (1973b) explained were characteristics of an object that are not presented directly but even so are there and add to the experience of the thing. He called this aspect of experience "apperceptions": When we grasp an object, we integrate apperceptions with what is actually presented before us. What we do not immediately and concretely experience are ap-perceived.

MARTIN HEIDEGGER

Heidegger was a student of Husserl, but Heidegger's philosophy of phenomenology did not focus on epistemological questions as his professor's did. Epistemology is the branch of philosophy that deals with the nature of knowledge. Heidegger's central concern was the ontological priority of the question of Being. Ontology is the branch of philosophy focusing on the nature of being. The question to be asked is about the meaning of Being. He used the term being-in-the-world to highlight the intertwined relationship between human existence and the world. What makes human beings different from other beings is their ability to be concerned about their very own being, which Heidegger termed "Dasein." He went on to say that being-in-the-world belongs essentially to Da-sein. Da-sein understands its own being in its close relationship with the world. Temporality is a fundamental aspect of Heidegger's philosophy of phenomenology. He argued that time is how Da-sein understands and interprets anything. Da-sein finds its meaning in temporality.

For Husserl, description was critical, while for Heidegger (1992), inter-pretation was critical, as he professed that it was the basic form for knowing. Interpretation (hermeneutics) was seen as critical for understanding because it helped disclose what is hidden or concealed. The primary work of phenom-enology is to lay open a phenomenon and let it be seen (Heidegger, 1992). Phenomena can be covered up in various ways. One way is that it is undis-covered. We have no knowledge of it and do not know it exists. Being buried is another way of being covered up. Here the phenomenon was earlier dis-covered but has gotten covered up. Disguise according to Heidegger (1992) is the most common and dangerous concealment. Here "the originally seen phenomena are uprooted, torn from their ground, and are no longer under-stood in their origins, in their 'extraction' from their roots in a particular subject matter" (p. 87). "Phenomenology means to let what shows itself be seen from itself, just as it shows itself from itself. That is the formal meaning of the type of research that calls itself phenomenology. But this expresses nothing other than the maxim formulated above: 'To the Things Themselves'!" (Heidegger, 1996, p. 30).

MAURICE MERLEAU-PONTY

Merleau-Ponty's philosophy of phenomenology is more an existential phenom-enology where "the world is always already there before reflection begins" (1996, p. vii) as opposed to Husserl's transcendental phenomenology. In *Phenomenology of Perception* (1996), Merleau-Ponty posited that "Perception is not a science of the world, it is not even an act, a deliberate taking up of a position; it is the background from which all acts stand out, and is presupposed by them" (p. x–xi). Merleau-Ponty attempted to bring the world of perception back to life. He declared that the world is hidden from us underneath all knowledge and social living. He also called for the need to return to things themselves prior to our knowledge.

Merleau-Ponty (1996) asserted that Fink, the assistant of Husserl, pro-vided the best view of reduction when Fink described that we must be aston-ished before the world. For Merleau-Ponty (1996), when practicing reflection, we do not withdraw from the world. Reflection "steps back to watch the forms of transcendence fly up like sparks from a fire; it slackens the intentional threads which attach us to the world as these bring them to our notice" (p. xiii). As Merleau-Ponty (1956) explained, complete reduction is not possible.

Merleau-Ponty's (1996) philosophy of phenomenology focused on put-ting back essences into experiences by not viewing them from theories or causal explanations. Merleau-Ponty (1956) warned that phenomenology is a laborious work due to the necessary attention, wonder, and demands of con-sciousness. For the philosopher, our bodies and the world are intertwined.

We live in both space and time. We have a temporal and spacial relationship with the world. In the *Visible and the Invisible,* Merleau-Ponty (1968) emphasized the flesh of the world. The importance of language permeates Merleau-Ponty's philosophy. In the *Prose of the World* (1973), he explained that "rather than imprisoning it, language is like a magic machine for transporting the 'I' into the other person's perspective" (p. 19).

HANS-GEORG GADAMER

Hans-Georg Gadamer studied under Heidegger. Gadamer's philosophy of phenomenology is essentially interpretive. It focuses on the explication of texts and not directly on the lived experience. His philosophy is based on human understanding. He emphasized that interpretation depends on a horizon of interpretation where understanding of a text occurs by a fusion of horizons: The horizon of the text and that of the person interpreting the text. In *Truth and Method,* Gadamer (2004) explained: "To acquire a horizon means that one learns to look beyond what is close at hand—not in order to look away from it but to see it better, within a larger whole and in truer proportion" (p. 304).

Gadamer stressed that the lifeworld is "the whole in which we live as historical creatures" (2004, p. 239). Openness is necessary to see the "otherness" of something. Tradition and historicity are part of the lifeworld. For Gadamer, meaning comes from both the past and also the present and even the future. Interpretation includes the historical context, both past and present. To achieve understanding, the interpreter moves between past and present and moves back and forth between parts of the text and the whole. For Gadamer, understanding takes place where tradition, the past, and the present intersect. Understanding includes prejudices that Gadamer explained are the results of the history of effect. Both prejudices and traditions occur in our understanding and hinder complete openness. We can increase our horizons of meaning when we overcome prejudices. Art is another component in Gadamer's (1998) hermeneutics. He explained that art can provide us with experiences that lead to new understanding of the world. When we place art in our historical and cultural lifeworld, it can provide us with understanding and an experience of truth.

In summary Husserl, Heidegger, Merleau-Ponty, and Gadamer's philosophies of phenomenology were briefly described to provide the foundation for the different descriptive and interpretive phenomenological methodologies that are covered in the remaining chapters of this book. Next in Chapter 3 Paul Colaizzi's methodology takes center stage and is the first of five descriptive phenomenological approaches that are addressed in Part II.

REFERENCES

Gadamer, H. G. (1998). *The relevance of the beautiful and other essays* (N. Walker, Trans.). Cambridge, UK: Cambridge University Press.

Gadamer, H. G. (2004). *Truth and method* (2nd Revision). (J. Weinsheimer & D. G. Marshall, Trans.). London: Continuum.

Heidegger, M. (1992). *History of the concept of time* (T. Kisiel, Trans.). Bloomington, IN: Indiana University Press.

Heidegger, M. (1996). *Being and time* (J. Stambaugh, Trans.). Albany, NY: State University of New York Press.

Husserl, E. (1931). *Ideas: General introduction to pure phenomenology.* (W. R. Boyce Gibson, Trans.). New York, NY: Collier Books.

Husserl, E. (1970). *The crisis of European sciences and transcendental phenomenology* (D. Carr, Trans.). Evanston, IL: Northwestern University Press.

Husserl, E. (1973a). *Cartesian meditations. An introduction to phenomenology* (D. Cairns, Trans.). The Hague, Netherlands: Martinus Nijhoff Publisher.

Husserl, E. (1973b). *Experience and judgment* (J. S. Churchill & K. Ameriks, Trans.). Evanston, IL: Northwestern University Press.

Husserl, E. (1981). Phenomenology and anthropology. In P. McCormick & F. Elliston (Eds.), *Husserl: Shorter works* (pp. 315–323) (R. G. Schmitt, Trans.). Notre Dame, IN: University of Notre Dame.

Husserl, E. (1983). *Ideas pertaining to a pure phenomenology and to a phenomenological philosophy* (D. Carr, Trans.). First Book: The Hague: Martinus Nijhoff Publisher. (F. Kersten, Trans.). Evanston, IL: Northwestern University Press.

Merleau-Ponty, M. (1956). What is phenomenology? *Cross-Currents, 34,* 59–70.

Merleau-Ponty, M. (1968). *The visible and the invisible* (A. Lingis, Trans.). Evanston, IL: Northwestern University Press.

Merleau-Ponty, M. (1996). *Phenomenology of perception* (C. Smith, Trans.). New York, NY: Routledge.

Merleau-Ponty, M. (1973). *The prose of the world* (J. O'Neill, Trans.). Evanston, IL: Northwestern University Press.

PART II

Descriptive Phenomenology

Paul Colaizzi's Descriptive Phenomenological Methodology

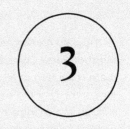

3

Paul Colaizzi's (1973, 1978) methodology of descriptive phenomenology is the focus of this chapter. His methodology is the first of three phenomenological approaches developed at Duquesne University linked to psychology. Giorgi and van Kaam's methodologies will be described in Chapters 4 and 5, respectively. First, the steps involved in conducting a study using his approach are described. An example of using Colaizzi's methodology is included from my program of research on postpartum depression. Next examples of studies incorporating Colaizzi's approach by researchers from a variety of disciplines are presented for illustration. These disciplines include Nursing, Public Health, Physiotherapy, Rehabilitation Therapy, Social Work, Occupational Therapy, and Psychology. These researchers provided an international use of Colaizzi's approach from the countries of United States, Iran, Canada, Australia, Spain, India, and Italy.

In Colaizzi's methodology, researchers begin by examining their presuppositions about the phenomenon being studied. He called for researchers to interrogate their beliefs, attitudes, hypotheses, and hunches regarding the phenomenon in order to discover them. Some questions that one can ask are "Why am I involved with this phenomenon? How might my personal inclinations and predisposition as to the research value influence or even bias how and what I investigate?" (1978, p. 55). An example of researchers examining their presuppositions comes from one of my phenomenological studies on postpartum depression. I kept a file on my computer where I described my preconceived beliefs about this mood disorder, knowledge I had of it from my literature reviews, and my clinical experiences as a nurse-midwife caring for new mothers suffering with this devastating psychiatric illness. I periodically updated this file with any new beliefs, attitudes, etc. Prior to interviewing participants for this study and during data analysis, I would reread what I had written in this file so my preconceived notions were front and center in my mind to help bracket them.

How do researchers know when they have eliminated their contaminating thoughts? Colaizzi supports Merleau-Ponty's (1956) belief that a complete reduction of all presuppositions is not possible. One can never totally guarantee that the researcher has successfully bracketed. What is required, though, is a change in the researcher's attitude so that the researcher can be present to the participant's experience. Colaizzi suggests that researchers can next compare their presuppositions with those of other persons. This comparison may help inform researchers of some additional presuppositions they may have passed over.

Bracketing is a challenge for researchers. It is a process and not something that can be done in one day or at one sitting. Researchers can keep a journal of their experiences, biases, and presuppositions about the phenomenon under study. Each day more entries can be made to the journal as researchers continually identify more information to put aside and bracket. Bracketing is done prior to collecting data with each participant and during data analysis so that the researchers' beliefs do not influence the research process. As data collection proceeds, researchers have more to bracket. Each participant's description of the experience being studied needs to be bracketed prior to interviewing the next participant.

....

RESEARCH QUESTION

A typical research question for a study using Colaizzi's methodology can be written as "What is the meaning of the experience of . . . ?" or "What is the essential structure of the experience of . . . ?" Researchers' interrogated presuppositions can be used by researchers to help formulate their research questions. The success of research questions depends on the degree to which they tap the participants' experiences of the phenomenon under study.

SAMPLE

Colaizzi (1978) offered the following criteria for sample inclusion: (1) The person has experience with the phenomenon under study and (2) the person can articulate that experience. A sample need not comprise a set number of participants. The sample size varies depending on various factors such as how rich the data are that each participant shares. Colaizzi gave a suggestion of 12 participants as an average number.

DATA COLLECTION

Colaizzi (1978) offered three options for collecting data in a phenomenological study. The first option is to ask for written protocols where the participants write down their experience. Colaizzi identified interviewing as another way to obtain data. Interviews need to be tape-recorded and transcribed. He calls these interviews dialogue interviews. Colaizzi explained that dialogue interviews can yield richer data than written data, which require the researcher to attend to the participants' nuances of speech and nonverbal behavior. During the interview, the researcher needs to engage in imaginative listening. Colaizzi emphasized that researchers must be present in a unique way during the interviews. Researchers need to listen to their participants with more than just their ears. They need to be totally present. Dialogic interviews need to occur in an environment of trust. If an interview is to be dialogal, it must take place among individuals on equal levels without diversification of professional or social stratifications. Colaizzi argued for dispensing with the strata of researchers and participants and instead referring to both as coresearchers.

The third type of phenomenological data collection for Colaizzi focuses on observations of lived events and perceptual description. Through observation, the researcher can investigate phenomena that cannot be communicated. In order to describe our observations, we must "describe what we see and not what we think we see" (Colaizzi, 1978, p. 65). Researchers need to eliminate contaminating thoughts in order to return to what they really observe. The method of perceptual description is what Colaizzi aligns with observation of lived events. Here instead of summarizing discrete perceptual facts, which leads to a perceptions of isolated things, the researcher strives for a perception of worlds.

DATA ANALYSIS

Colaizzi's (1978) steps of the data analysis process can be found in Figure 3.1, which I had created for my study on the impact of birth trauma on breastfeeding (Beck & Watson, 2008). Colaizzi alerted potential users of his approach that there is often overlapping of the steps and that the sequences should be considered flexible. After collecting the data, the researcher reads and rereads the transcripts. Next, significant statements are extracted from the participants' descriptions of the phenomenon under study. If transcripts contain the same or merely identical significant statements, these replications can be eliminated. The next step, known as formulating meanings, is where the researcher takes a "precarious leap" from what the participants say to what

FIGURE 3.1

Colaizzi's Procedure Steps for Analyzing Data Phenomenologically

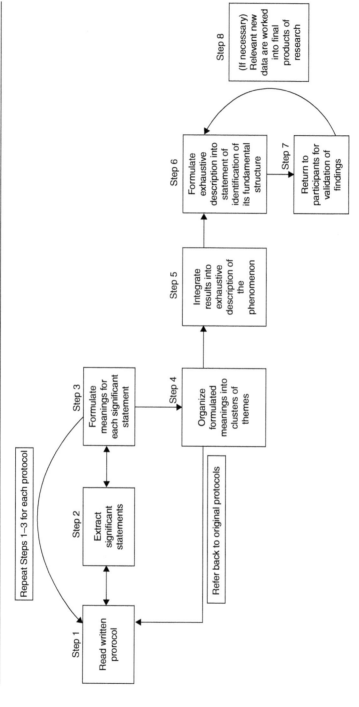

Source: Reprinted with permission from Beck, C. T., & Watson, S. (2008). The impact of birth trauma on breastfeeding: A tale of two pathways. *Nursing Research, 57*, 228–236. p. 231.

they mean. Formulated meanings should never cut all connection with the original description by the participant. In this step, the researcher is trying to discover hidden meanings that are contained in the original protocols. Colaizzi (1978) stated that

> contextual and horizontal meanings are given with the protocol but are not in it; so the researcher must go beyond what is given in the original data and at the same time, stay with it. He must not formulate meanings which have no connection with the data. (p. 59)

He insisted that researchers must not impose any theories on the data and instead must allow the data to speak for themselves. "The investigator, in order to objectively articulate the meaning of the data, must remain alert to avoid projecting subjective meanings into the data that ultimately originate in, and would artificially confirm, his research purpose" (Colaizzi, 1973, pp. 113–114).

The formulated meanings are next sorted into clusters of themes. These clusters are then referred back to the original protocols to validate them. If the themes are not validated, then the researcher must reexamine or reconduct the prior steps. The researcher at this point should "rely upon his tolerance for ambiguity" (Colaizzi, 1978, p. 61), as discrepancies may be noted among themes. The researcher needs to refuse the temptation to remove some data or themes that don't seem to really fit. Once the themes are validated with the original transcripts, now the researcher integrates the results so far into an exhaustive description of the phenomenon being studied. After this is written, the exhaustive description is formulated into an unequivocal statement that identifies the fundamental structure. Lastly, a validating step can be done where the researcher returns to the participants to ask "How do my descriptive results compare with your experiences? What aspects of your experience or of your existence have I omitted?" (Colaizzi, 1978, p. 62). Any relevant data given by the participants are worked into the final outcome of the research. Validating their first draft of the fundamental structure with participants in the study helps researchers be confident they have adequately identified the fundamental structure of the experience being studied.

THE LIVED EXPERIENCE OF POSTPARTUM DEPRESSION

In this section, I have chosen to illustrate Colaizzi's approach by describing one of my phenomenological studies on the essential structure of the experience of postpartum depression (Beck, 1992). A purposive sample of seven women who had suffered from postpartum depression participated in in-depth interviews. Before each interview, I bracketed my experiences as a certified nurse-midwife who cared for mothers suffering with this postpartum mood disorder. Each recorded interview started with the statement: Please describe for me your experiences of postpartum depression. Share all your thoughts, feelings, and perceptions that you can recall until you have no more to say. Any specific examples of points that you are making will be extremely valuable.

After transcribing the interviews, significant statements about postpartum depression were extracted and formulated meanings were made for each statement. Table 3.1 provides selected examples of significant statements and their corresponding formulated meanings. Next I clustered the formulated meanings into themes (Table 3.2). From this process, 11 themes emerged, and an exhaustive description of the experience of postpartum depression was given to three of the seven mothers to review. Two mothers suggested that I needed to stress more their self-hatred for being a failure as a mother and also their becoming a hypochondriac. These two points were added, and the final fundamental structure of postpartum depression was developed (Table 3.3).

TABLE 3.1

Selected Examples of Significant Statements of Postpartum Depression and Corresponding Formulated Meanings

Significant Statements	Formulated Meanings
I obsessed all day long with what's wrong with me.	The mother was filled with obsessive thoughts throughout the day questioning what was wrong with her.
My biggest fear was that I wasn't going to get better and that I wasn't going to be the same person I was.	What the mother feared the most was that she would never get better and never be the same person she had been before the postpartum depression.
It was like a withdrawal of emotions. I felt as if I was acting; I went through the motions of my life without any of the joy.	The mother described feeling like she was acting and just went through the motions of her life without any joy.

Source: Author Created.

TABLE 3.2

Examples of Two Theme Clusters With Their Subsumed Formulated Meanings

The mother envisioned herself as a robot stripped of all feelings, just going through the motions.

a. She would just go through the mechanics when caring for her baby.
b. Feelings of emptiness prevailed.
c. She was unable to feel any emotions.
d. She felt like a robot who just went through the motions.
e. Sheer exhaustion left the mother with nothing to give herself or her baby.

Shrouded in fogginess, the mother's ability to concentrate diminished.

a. She felt as if she was drifting in a fog with her mind filled with cobwebs.
b. Attempts to overcome the depression were hindered by the fogginess and fatigue.
c. Loss of both concentration and sometimes motor skills occurred.
d. She experienced being in a totally different dimension.

Source: Reprinted with permission from Beck, C. T. (1992). The lived experience of postpartum depression: A phenomenological study. *Nursing Research, 41*, 166–170. p. 168.

TABLE 3.3

Fundamental Structure of Postpartum Depression

Postpartum depression is a living nightmare in which death is contemplated as the ultimate escape. Severe, uncontrollable anxiety drives the mother to becoming a hypochondriac and imprint in her an aura of teetering on the edge of insanity. Loss of control over one's emotions prevails as overwhelming insecurities suffocate independence. Obsessive thoughts of failure as a mother and questioning what is wrong with her bombard a mother's waking hours. All-consuming guilt and fear, leading to self-hate, are experienced as the horror of thoughts of harming the infant are pondered. Enveloped in loneliness, a mother's life is further compromised by a void of all previous interests and goals. Concentration level is severely diminished as fogginess sets in. Postpartum depression is associated with a vision of self as a robot devoid of all feelings just going through the motions. While grieving the loss of self, fear is all-encompassing as one envisions that prior normalcy in her life is irretrievable.

Source: Reprinted with permission from Beck, C. T., & Watson, S. (2010). Subsequent childbirth after a previous traumatic birth. *Nursing Research, 59*, 241–249. p. 245.

EXAMPLES OF RESEARCH FROM VARIOUS DISCIPLINES

In Iran from the discipline of Public Health, health care managers' experiences in providing nutritional aid during an earthquake were investigated (Moghadam, Amiresmaieli, Hassibi, Doostan, & Khosravi, 2017). Ten male managers were interviewed, and Colaizzi's approach resulted in four themes and 19 subthemes regarding challenges in the nutritional aid during the Bam Earthquake. The main issues in distributing foodstuffs for the disaster-stricken people included managerial problems, nutritional problems, infrastructural problems, and administrative problems. Each main issue consisted of secondary issues. For example, for the main issue of nutritional problems, the secondary issues were quality food, unfamiliarity with the nutritional needs of the population, lack of attention to the food variety sent to the victims, and inconsistency between foreign foods and the Iranian culture.

The experience of heterotopic ossification in adults following a burn was the topic of a phenomenological study in Australia from the discipline of Physiotherapy (Foster, Kornhaber, McGarry, Wood, & Edgar, 2017). Knowledge of burn survivors' experiences of this severely debilitating complication helped to gain a greater understanding of the clinical needs of these patients. Using Colaizzi's steps to analyze interviews of five men and one woman yielded five themes: Early signs and symptoms, Impact on the rehabilitation journey, Role of the health care professionals, Loss of independence and an increased reliance on others, and Learning to live with it: uncertainty, hope and adaptation.

In Canada from Rehabilitation Therapy, Marshall, Lysaght and Krupa (2017) examined the experiences of occupational engagement of chronically homeless people in a midsized urban context. Using purposive sampling, 12 persons who had been homeless continuously for 1 year or 4 times in the past 3 years were selected for interviews. Colaizzi's (1978) steps of phenomenological analysis yielded five themes: Occupational alienation, Getting a different feeling, Negotiating the social context, Taking care of others, and Every day is about trying to survive.

In Italy, nurse researchers explored the experiences of older persons following an acute exacerbation of chronic obstructive pulmonary disease (COPD) (Rosa et al., 2018). In-depth interviews were conducted with 12 patients recovering from an acute exacerbation of COPD. Using Colaizzi's steps in data analysis, first significant statements were extracted from the interview transcripts and meanings were formulated. An example of one significant statement was,

> But I tell you that I'm a little worried because I worry about going back home, but not from the financial point of view, just from the standpoint of what I will do and how I will face life in this way, you know. (p. e1113)

The meaning formulated from this significant statement was, "He is worried about the future. He seems to despair about his life from now on" (p. e1113). Next the researchers clustered formulated meanings into themes. For the theme of Fear of becoming a burden, an example of two formulated meanings clustered together was, "He feels like an inconvenience or burden. He is aware that his family have busy lives to explain and excuse their lack of help for him" (p. e1114). Further analysis revealed four themes: Sense of loss and frustration, Hopelessness, Uncertainly about the future, and Fear of becoming a burden.

Challenges for family caregivers of young adults with traumatic brain injuries as they transition from pediatric to adult services were explored in Canada by social work researchers (Shankar et al., 2018). Their research question was "What are the lived experiences and challenges faced by family caregivers as they help their young adult traumatic brain injury survivor transition to services and supports for adults?" (p. 2). Fifteen family caregivers were interviewed, and the data they provided were analyzed using Colaizzi's (1978) methodology. Shankar and colleagues identified 85 significant statements that were clustered into 15 themes. Examples of significant statements with their corresponding formulated meanings were included in their article. Also examples of two themes with their formulated meanings were provided to illustrate these steps. For instance for the theme of Difficulty getting information about available services, one formulated meaning subsumed under it was "The parent is frustrated at the lack of honest answers from service providers" (p. 4). Some selected themes from the list of 15 themes were:

- Concerns about loss of peer relationships

- Working proactively with their child

- Expectations versus reality

- Racism and discrimination

- Conflicting information

Occupational therapists in Iran described the experience of living with chronic insomnia using Colaizzi's (1978) methodology (Rezaie, Khazaie, & Yazdani, 2016). The sample consisted of 15 participants (8 females and 7 males). After bracketing, each interview began with these statements: "Please tell me about your experience of insomnia" and "Please tell me how you live with insomnia" (p. 180). Analysis revealed 180 significant statements that were clustered into two themes: (1) Upset mind and (2) Unwanted new lifestyle. As part of Colaizzi's methodology, Rezaie et al. wrote up an exhaustive description of the phenomenon. They shared the themes, subthemes, and exhaustive description with the participants to validate their findings. All the participants agreed with the results. The first theme of Upset mind had two subthemes of Insomnia as an unpleasant experience and Insomnia as a worrying experience. The second theme of Unwanted new lifestyle included three subthemes: (1) Treatment seeking behavior, (2) Boring new daily routine, and (3) Being overshadowed by depressed mood. The researchers included examples of formulated meanings for the themes. Some formulated meanings that were clustered under the theme of Unwanted new lifestyle were "experience of sadness, crying, irritability, loss of energy, lack of interest in participating in social interaction, and lack of warmth with family" (Rezaie et al., 2016, p. 181).

In summary, the steps involved in Paul Colaizzi's descriptive phenomenological methodology were explained in this chapter. From around the globe, cross-disciplinary examples of research using his approach were included as illustrations. In Appendices A and B can be found study activities for students. Next in Chapter 4 the second descriptive phenomenological methodology, that of Amedeo Giorgi, is addressed.

REFERENCES

Beck, C. T. (1992). The lived experience of postpartum depression: A phenomenological study. *Nursing Research, 41*, 166–170.

Beck, C. T., & Watson, S. (2008). The impact of birth trauma on breastfeeding: A tale of two pathways. *Nursing Research, 57*, 228–236.

Colaizzi, P. H. (1973). *Reflection and research in psychology: A phenomenological study of learning.* Dubuque, IA: Kendall/Hunt Publishing Company.

Colaizzi, P. H. (1978). Psychological research as the phenomenologist views it. In R. S. Valle & M. King (Eds.), *Existential phenomenological alternatives for psychology* (pp. 48–71). New York, NY: Oxford University Press.

Foster, N., Kornhaber, R., McGarry, S., Wood, F. M., & Edgar, D. W. (2017). Heterotopic ossification in adults following a burn: A phenomenological analysis. *Burns, 43*, 1250–1262.

Marshall, C. A., Lysaght, R., & Krupa, T. (2017). The experience of occupational engagement of chronically homeless persons in a mid-sized urban context. *Journal of Occupational Science, 24*, 165–180.

Merleau-Ponty, M. (1956). What is phenomenology? *Cross-Currents, 34*, 59–70.

Moghadam, M. N., Amiresmaiele, M., Hassibi, M., Doostan, F., & Khosravi, S. (2017). Toward a better nutritional aiding in disasters: Relying on lessons learned during the Bam Earthquake. *Prehospital and Disaster Medicine, 32*, 382–386.

Rezaie, L., Khazaie, H., & Yazdani, F. (2016). Exploration of the experience of living with chronic insomnia: A qualitative study. *Sleep Science, 9*, 179–185.

Rosa, F., Bagnasco, A., Ghirotto, L., Rocco, G., Catania, G., Aleo, G., Zanini, M., Dasso, N., Hayter, M., & Sasso, L. (2018). Experiences of older people following an acute exacerbation of chronic obstructive pulmonary disease: A phenomenological study. *Journal of Clinical Nursing, 27*, e1110–1119.

Shankar, J., Nicholas, D., Mrazik, M., Waugh, E., Tan, S., Zulla, R., Urichuk, L., & Paranica, S. (2018). Transition from pediatric to adult services: Challenges for family caregivers of young adults with traumatic brain injury. *Sage Open*, October-December, 1–14. doi: 10.1177/215824407954

Amedeo Giorgi's Descriptive Phenomenological Methodology

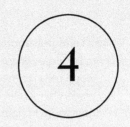

In this chapter, Amedeo Giorgi's descriptive phenomenological methodology takes center stage. It is the second approach developed at Duquesne University to be addressed in this book. The steps that make up his approach are each addressed. Giorgi's study on jealousy is used to illustrate his process. Examples of research using his methodology are described, including studies from Sweden, Ireland, Korea, and Spain, representing the disciplines of Nursing, Psychology, English, and Education.

In Giorgi's (2009) descriptive phenomenological approach, the researcher first begins by assuming the correct attitude, that being the attitude of phenomenological reduction. When researchers assume this attitude, they take what is given in their consciousness as a presence, not an existence. Giorgi's approach, based directly on Husserl's philosophy (1983), focuses on the description of a phenomenon from within the reduction so as to uncover the essence of a phenomenon with the aid of free imagination. Giorgi does not call for just one level of Husserl's reduction. The first level involves the object presented to consciousness being understood as something that is present as it is experienced and not a claim of its existence exactly as it is experienced. The second level of phenomenological reduction focuses on bracketing, or also called epoché, of prior knowledge or presuppositions about the given object. Giorgi (2009) explains that though the word *reduction* implies a cutting back, in phenomenology it instead provides a heightening of the researcher's presence in the activity of consciousness. Bracketing allows the researcher's attention to focus on the present experience. It is not a matter of the researcher's forgetting past experiences but instead of not permitting past knowledge to color what participants are describing. It allows researchers to be critically attentive to the experiences of the participant. In practicing epoché, it is helpful for researchers to find a quiet place to reflect on their past experiences, thoughts, and feelings. Multiple sessions are needed until the researchers feel they have brought their biases and presuppositions into their consciousness. It allows the research-ers to be more receptive to listening to what participants say.

Giorgi calls for the use of Husserl's free imaginative variation, which helps the researcher achieve a higher level of invariant meaning or essence of the phenomenon. Imaginative variation involves a process of reflective phases where researchers examine many different possibilities and use different frames of reference and divergent perspectives in an attempt to identify essential meanings of the experience under study. In free imaginative varia-tion, the researcher mentally removes an aspect of the phenomenon under study to determine if this removal transforms the description in an essen-tial way. If so, this leans toward its being essential to the phenomenon. An example of the use of free imaginative variation can be illustrated by a lamp. If the lampshade were removed, it would still be a lamp, but if the socket were removed, it would no longer be a lamp. Giorgi prefers the language of structure instead of essence because most often there are multiple key invariant meanings for each phenomenological study. Structure refers to the relationship among these invariant meanings.

Giorgi (2014) called for a phenomenological methodology where there is a transformation of the participant's data, but these are clarifying transforma-tions intrinsic to the participant's description. The context of these transfor-mations is provided by the participant's own perspective. These meanings are clarified without the use of any theories. According to Giorgi, his approach makes explicit the psychological meaning expressed by the participants.

In Giorgi's methodology, he uses psychology to provide an example of his phenomenological approach since psychology is his discipline. Giorgi (2012) makes it clear, however, that his phenomenological approach is generic enough to be applied to any social science discipline such as Sociology or Education. The only change would be that researchers assume the attitude of their discipline instead of a psychological attitude.

RESEARCH QUESTION

A typical research question using Giorgi's approach would be written as "What is the general structure of the phenomenon . . . ?"

SAMPLE

In Giorgi's (2009) methodology, at least three participants are necessary for a phenomenological sample. The number of participants, however, depends on the amount of raw data collected from each person. What is counted is not the number of participants, but instead the number of instances of the phenomenon being studied that are contained in the participants' descriptions of their experiences. The more data participants share about their experience, the smaller the sample size needed. Giorgi reminds researchers that they are seeking the structure of a phenomenon and not the individualized experience.

DATA COLLECTION

Giorgi explains that one criterion for a phenomenological interview that a researcher needs is to have as complete a description as possible of the experience being studied that a participant has lived through. During the interview, the researcher puts aside any past experiences or any favorite theories in order not to be tempted by them when exploring the participant's experience.

DATA ANALYSIS

The steps in Giorgi's (2009) descriptive phenomenological approach in psychology, which he called a modified Husserlian approach, are as follows:

1. Read for sense of the whole.

   When reading all the transcribed descriptions of the phenomenon under study, the researcher assumes the attitude of the scientific phenomenological reduction. Giorgi (2012) describes a psychological perspective, but he notes that the perspective depends on the researcher's discipline.

2. Determination of meaning units.

   In this step, the entire description being analyzed is broken into meaning units so that each passage is given its due attention. Meaning units help researchers focus on the parts of the whole description so a detailed analysis is possible. Giorgi (2014) explains that this is a practical step for descriptions. Meaning units are divisions in the transcripts where a significant shift in meaning occurs. Giorgi (2009) emphasizes that meaning units do not carry theoretical weight. These units are just the result of making the original descriptions of the phenomenon more manageable. Not every researcher who identifies meaning units in the same transcript will delineate the same meaning units. What is important is how the meaning units are transformed and integrated into the structure of the phenomenon under study. All of the meaning units are interdependent. They do not exist alone, as the whole description is taken into account. Giorgi (2014) bases this on Husserl's (1970) philosophy of the relationship between parts and wholes. Independent parts can stand alone, but dependent parts cannot. Husserl called dependent parts, moments. Giorgi states that his meaning units are these moments since they are interdependent. For Giorgi (2006), the meaning units are delineated. No part of the entire description is left out. Giorgi does not want to decontextualize the statement. Redundancies are kept so as to keep the entire description. In description, researchers acknowledge that there is a given that they need to describe as it appears without adding or subtracting anything external to the data. Researchers do not adopt a non-given factor, such as a theory, hypothesis, or assumption, to help account for what is given in the experience (Giorgi, 2012).

3. Transformation of participants' natural attitude expressions into phenomenologically psychologically sensitive expressions.

This third step is the heart of Giorgi's approach. It is, however, the most challenging one. Each meaning unit is interrogated in order to identify its psychological implications for the description. These second order descriptions are invariant meanings in which the researcher uses free imaginative variation. Invariant meanings constitute structures that have the strength of facts. The researcher imagines how the data are different from what they are to find higher level categories that keep the same psychological meaning but are not embedded in the same described situation. Giorgi is well aware that every participant's description of an experience will be different from that of other participants. However, the psychological meaning can be the same even if the facts differ. The psychosocial meanings researchers are searching for reach a level of invariance that can comprehend multiple, different facts. In this step, the phenomenologists try to generalize the data so it is easier for them to integrate findings from various participants into one general structure of the phenomenon under study.

Giorgi (2009) suggests using two to three columns to help transform meaning units more explicitly in language revelatory of the psychological aspect. Not every meaning unit necessarily has the same number of transformations. The first column just repeats the exact words of the participants with one minor change. Now everything is changed into third-person instead of first-person expressions. Giorgi claims that this change is important to make clear phenomenologists are analyzing another's experiences and not their own. In the second column, researchers try to describe the psychological senses that present themselves to their consciousness.

TABLE 4.1

Example of Three Columns Used in Giorgi's Analysis of the Description of Jealousy

P_2 and Pam are both in the fifth grade in a little country school with six grades and only 62 students. They are not friends or enemies.	P_2 describes the circumstances of their acquaintanceship. She and the person who is the object of her attention are in the same grade in a small, country school and P_2 states that she and her classmate are neither very close nor at odds with each other but merely acquaintances.	P_2 explains the nature of the acquaintanceship that exists between herself and her ideal, which is distant familiarity and not overtly antagonistic.

Source: Reprinted with permission from Giorgi, A. (2009). *The descriptive phenomenological method in Psychology: A modified Husserlian Approach.* Pittsburgh, PA: Duquesne University Press. pp. 157–158.

The first transformed meaning that comes to mind may not be the best one. A third column is then needed to ensure some generalization because it is assumed that each description of the phenomenon under study is different from every other one. Generalizing meaning units helps to integrate results across participants. Transformed meaning units provide the basis for writing the general structure of the phenomenon. Table 4.1 provides an example of these three columns provided by Giorgi (2009, pp. 157–158) for a description of jealousy.

4. Writing the general structure

This final step involves a more holistic approach reviewing all the last transformed meaning units in the 2nd and 3rd columns for all the participants. This is done in order to compare and contrast them. What are the key constituent meanings of the phenomenon, and what are the relationships among them? To determine if a constituent meaning is a key of a general structure is to see if the structure collapses if it is deleted. Giorgi (2009) specified that a constituent differs from an element. An element is a part that is independent of the whole where it resides. A constituent, however, is a part related to its role in the whole. So for Giorgi in developing a general structure of a phenomenon, the researcher focuses on the relationship among the identified constituents. Below is the general structure of Giorgi's study of jealousy:

> Jealousy is experienced in a situation where P is not receiving sufficient attention and appreciation for herself and another person actively robs P of the already lacking attention and appreciation desired by P. Intense feelings of resentment and hostility towards the other is experienced when the other seems to take advantage of an unfair privileged position and uses this privilege to undermine P's position and P's possibility to attain the attention she seeks. P finds these negative strong emotions and physical responses uncomfortable and P intensely wishes to hide her responses from others. (Giorgi, 2009, p. 179)

As you have read in the previous chapter, Colaizzi (1978) called for returning to the coresearchers to validate the exhaustive description of the phenomenon being studied. Giorgi (1989) has an opposite view of this practice. He asserts that there is not a problem with the researcher returning to subjects to ask them to clarify a point in their original description. It is not appropriate, however, to ask subjects to evaluate the researcher's findings since they have been analyzed from a psychological perspective. Giorgi further declares that having subjects evaluate the results exceeds their role as subjects.

EXAMPLES OF PUBLISHED STUDIES USING GIORGI'S DESCRIPTIVE PHENOMENOLOGICAL METHODOLOGY

Lindberg, Fagerström, Willman, and Sivberg (2017) used Giorgi's phenomenological approach to investigate the meaning of being an autonomous person while dependent on advanced medical technology at home. The lead researcher is from the Department of Health at the Blekinge Institute of Technology in Sweden. The researchers said that, since a scientific perspective should be chosen for the analysis with the language specific to a discipline, they chose the scientific perspective of caring science. Lindberg and colleagues identified the constituents as (1) befriending the lived body, (2) depending on good relationships, (3) keeping the home as a private sphere, and (4) managing time. They developed a general structure of the meaning of being an autonomous person while dependent on advanced medical technology at home that was as follows:

> The lived body sets the boundaries for the life with advanced medical technology at home. Although enabling a sense of freedom, supporting

one's own existence through the generation of conditions for everyday life, the technology involved dependence and a vulnerability engendering ambivalent feelings. The technology exerted an influence, not only on the patients themselves but also on the everyday life of the entire family. The relationships with the staff required integrity and mutual responsibility, along with staff competence, accessibility, and continuity. Participation in decisions was preferable to a far too great self-determination, and by being an active agent, the worth as a person could be fostered. The home was the favored care environment even if this private sphere was challenged by the use of advanced medical technology. The health status and not the technology itself was the largest hindrance for inside and outside activities. Day and night use of technology created a need for flexibility of care hours in relation to everyday life. (Lindberg et al., 2017, p. 848)

Another example of researchers using Giorgi's approach comes from the discipline of Psychology. In Norway, Tangvald-Petersen and Bongaardt (2017) explored a sense of belonging in the workplace as experienced by 16 persons struggling with mental health issues. The researchers utilized Giorgi's steps of first reading the entire interview transcript and then dividing the text into manageable meaning units. As Giorgi (2009) suggested, they inserted slashes into the body of the text where there seemed to be a shift in focus. Free imaginative variation was used in analyzing the meaning units. Next a comprehensive description of the general structure of the lived experience of belonging in the workplace of persons with mental health problems was developed. Here is an excerpt from this structure:

A sense of belonging in the workplace starts to evolve from the moment one's colleagues choose to let one in. At this point, one's status changes from being a casual outcast to becoming a naturalized part of the community at work. Until such time as this happens, one is dead-locked in a position of insecurity and bewilderment. Working and not knowing whether one is inside or outside the working group generates a vigilant sensitivity towards colleagues and the workplace, which can very easily evolve into a thwarted sense of belonging or even prevent it from developing at all. (Tangvald-Petersen & Bongaardt, 2017, p. 4)

In the Republic of Korea, Kim (2017), a nurse researcher, examined the life experiences of positive growth in 15 long-term childhood cancer survivors. Kim conducted in-depth interviews using questions like "What are the positive aspects of your post-treatment life? What factors have affected your positive growth?" (p. 61). Using Giorgi's phenomenological approach, Kim identified meaning units from the interview transcripts, transformed them into psychological sensitive expressions, and then clustered them into themes. Table 4.2 provides examples of three steps in Giorgi's data analysis methodology that Kim employed.

Isabirye and Makoe (2018), representing the discipline of Education in South Africa, used Giorgi's methodology to explore the lived experiences of six academics who participated in a professional development program that focused on moving the faculty from traditional distance teaching to online facilitation

TABLE 4.2

Example From the Three Steps of Giorgi's Data Analysis Used by Kim

Participants description	Meaning unit	Transformation
Participant 5 says, "I think a normal life like everyone else has . . . like going to school, playing sports, hanging out with friends . . . things like that seem like positive growth. I have many things to do, and everything seems so fun." Participant 2 says, "I feel like blending in with other people and living like everyone else." Also, "During the treatment period, my relationship with my friends was severed. Thus, I think it's important to live well with others, like friends."	Participant reported that living a normal life similar to everyone else represents positive growth. Participant thought a normal life that also included building good relationships represents positive growth.	Participants placed significance on the ability to live a normal life "like everyone else." Their perceptions of a normal life also included building good relationships.

Source: Reprinted with permission from Kim, Y. (2017). Exploration of life experiences of positive growth in long-term childhood cancer survivors. *European Journal of Oncology Nursing, 30,* 60–66. p. 63.

of learning. After bracketing, the researchers conducted face-to-face interviews. The transcribed interviews were read to obtain a global sense. Then per Giorgi's approach, the raw data were divided into meaning units, translated into psychological language in the third person while keeping their central meaning. Eventually, the researchers developed a description of the structure of the experience of these six academics. Examples of their meaning units were provided such as, "We were told how important it was to use 'my Unisa' as a tool to facilitate online learning" and "the importance of facilitating learning in a more authentic, collaborative and interactive way" (Isabirye & Makoe, 2018, p. 4).

From the Department of English in Korea, Lee (2017) explored how three undergraduate university students experienced their peer assessment activities in interpreter education. In scale-referenced peer assessment, students assessed their peers' performances on a pre-specified rating scale. Lee collected data in three ways: students' reflective journals, interviews, and mind maps. Lee used Giorgi's steps in data processing. Table 4.3 provides an example of three

TABLE 4.3

Example of Three of Giorgi's Steps Lee Used

Step 3: Meaning units
Before the first training session, I presumed that we, non-expert raters, would assess the samples from different perspectives, leading to inter-rater disagreement. My assumption was not wrong, but inter-rater disagreement was much greater than I expected.
I also noticed that my scores were always (at least) two points below the average, so I carefully considered myself and the internal criteria by which I had rated interpretations. My self-reflection began with the following questions: Am I wrong? In what areas?

Step 4: General expressions restated in ordinary language
During the first training session, P3 discovered that differences in rating between students were much greater than initially expected.
P3 realized that she tended to assign lower scores than her peers to the same sample, so she reflected critically on herself as a rater.

Step 5: Shortened, synthesized descriptions
During the first training session, P3 discovered substantial inter-rater disagreement and reflected critically on herself as a rater.

Source: Reprinted with permission from Lee, S. B. (2017). University students' experience of scale-referenced peer assessment for a consecutive interpreting examination. *Assessment and Evaluation in Higher Education, 42,* 1015–1029. p. 1022.

of Giorgi's steps Lee used. Data analysis resulted in Lee identifying the general structure of undergraduate students' experiences of scale-referenced peer assessment in interpreting examination:

> For P (the three participants as a collective abbreviation), the experience of engaging in scale-referenced, summative peer assessment activities begins with expressing concern about peer assessment. P worries about (a) assigning scores to peer students in the examination, and (b) having to use a pre-specified rating scale for that. However, during peer assessment training sessions, P participates actively in peer assessment with a sense of responsibility, feeling as if P has become an interpreter trainer or an expert. Meanwhile, P is surprised to know that assessment results may be greatly different among assessors. P also realizes that rating interpretation performances against predetermined criteria is more challenging than initially expected. In particular, P feels that assessing more than 10 students on the rating scale within a time limit is an exhausting process. After the entire process, P becomes convinced that peer assessment is beneficial and reliable. However, P regrets not providing sufficient, substantive or positive feedback. (Lee, 2017, p. 1023)

In summary, Amedeo Giorgi's methodology of descriptive phenomenology was presented. International examples of studies conducted from various disciplines were included to help illustrate his approach. As a reminder, Appendices A and B have two student learning activities. Next in Chapter 5 the descriptive phenomenological methodology to be covered in this book is focused on, that being, Adrian van Kaam's approach and Moustakas's modification of it.

REFERENCES

Colaizzi, P. H. (1978). Psychological research as the phenomenologist views it. In R. S. Valle & M. King (Eds.), *Existential phenomenological alternatives for psychology* (pp. 48–71). New York, NY: Oxford University Press.

Giorgi, A. (1989). Some theoretical and practical issues regarding the psychological phenomenological method. *Saybrook Review, 7*, 71–85.

Giorgi, A. (2006). Concerning variations in the application of the phenomenological method. *The Humanistic Psychologist, 34*, 305–319.

Giorgi, A. (2009). *The descriptive phenomenological method in psychology: A modified Husserlian Approach*. Pittsburgh, PA: Duquesne University Press.

Giorgi, A. (2012). The descriptive phenomenological psychological method. *Journal of Phenomenological Psychology, 43*, 3–12.

Giorgi, A. (2014). An affirmation of the phenomenological psychological descriptive method: A response to Rennie (2012). *Psychological Methods, 13*, 542–551.

Husserl, E. (1970). *Logical investigations* (Vol. 2; J. N. Finlay, Trans.). New York, NY : Humanities Press.

Husserl, E. (1983). *Ideas pertaining to a pure phenomenology and to a phenomenological psychology* (F. Kersten, Trans.). The Hague: Nijhoff.

Isabirye, A. K., & Makoe, M. (2018). Phenomenological analysis of the lived experiences of academics who participated in the professional development programme at an open distance learning (ODL) University in South Africa. *The Indo-Pacific Journal of Phenomenology, 18*(1), 11pp. doi: 10.1080/20797222.2018.1450764

Kim, Y. (2017). Exploration of life experiences of positive growth in long-term childhood cancer survivors. *European Journal of Oncology Nursing, 30*, 60–66.

Lee, S. B. (2017). University students' experience of scale-referenced peer assessment for a consecutive interpreting examination. *Assessment & Evaluation in Higher Education, 42*, 1015–1029.

Lindberg, C., Fagerström, C., Willman, A., & Sivberg, B. (2017). Befriending everyday life when bringing technology into the private sphere. *Qualitative Health Research, 27*, 843–854.

Tangvald-Petersen, O., & Bongaardt, R. (2017). The interconnection between mental health, work, and belonging: A phenomenological investigation. *The Indo-Pacific Journal of Phenomenology, 17*(2), 11pp. doi: 10.1080/20797222.2017.1392759

Adrian van Kaam's Descriptive Phenomenological Methodology and Clark Moustakas's Modification

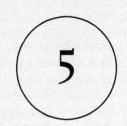

The focus of this chapter is Adrian van Kaam's (1966) descriptive phenomenological methodology. It is the third approach developed at Duquesne University. His approach has a bit of a quantitative feel to it because of his use of some quantitative terms such as random sample and explication. van Kaam's approach is explained, and examples of studies conducted in the United States and Australia are presented as an illustration. Also addressed in this chapter is Clark Moustakas's (1994) modification of van Kaam's approach. Selected examples from the disciplines of Business, Education, Social Work, Psychology, Nursing, and Information Technology are described.

van Kaam (1987) explained his purpose in developing his new phenomenological methodology in Psychology was to describe and analyze scientifically the psychological structures of experiences of humans. The structures of situated experiences as described by an intersubjectively verifiable methodology would, for van Kaam, provide the origin of data for Psychology. A basic assumption of van Kaam is that the core of common experiences is the same in different persons. The aim of his method is to identify the necessary and sufficient constituents of an experience. He defined a necessary constituent of a certain experience as "a moment of the experience which, while explicitly or implicitly expressed in a significant majority of explications by a random sample of subjects, is also compatible with those descriptions which do not express it" (van Kaam, 1983, p. 118). In van Kaam's approach, explication is central. In the process of explication, "implicit awareness of a complex phenomenon becomes explicit, formulated knowledge of its components" (van Kaam, 1966, p. 305). An enlightened awareness includes the necessary and sufficient constituents of the experiences that are precisely represented.

In describing his methodology, van Kaam did not specifically use the term "bracket" but did stress the researcher must restrict himself in his explication to the expression of what is given in awareness. "During the process of explication he ought not to involve himself in any implicit philosophizing, be he of a Freudian, a behavioristic, a stimulus-response, a Jungian, or any other school." (van Kaam, 1966, p. 306) He contended that researchers who begin with their own analyzed experience run the risk of being prejudiced from the start. No theoretical prejudice should be present.

RESEARCH QUESTION

An example of a typical research question in a study based on van Kaam's methodology is, "What are the necessary and sufficient constituents of the phenomenon of . . .?"

SAMPLE

van Kaam does not specify the required number of subjects needed in a sample. His approach though involves a larger sample than any of the other phenomenological methodologies. An indication of this large sample comes from this quote: "The scientist makes his initial categories from empirical data, in this case a sufficiently large random sample of cases taken from the total pool of descriptions" (van Kaam, 1966, pp. 314–315). An example of what van Kaam (1983) means by a large sample comes from his study on the experience of really feeling understood. In this sample, he collected data from 365 high school students.

van Kaam calls persons in a sample "subjects." This is in contrast to Colaizzi (1978), who calls participants "coresearchers." In choosing a sample, van Kaam (1966) identified key criteria. First of all the subjects have had the experience of the phenomenon being studied. Then he suggested these additional criteria:

a. The ability to express themselves with relative ease in the English language.

b. The ability to sense and to express inner feelings and emotions without shame and inhibition.

c. The ability to sense and to express the organic experiences that accompany these feelings.

d. A spontaneous interest in this experience on the part of the subject.

e. An atmosphere in which the subject can find the necessary relaxation to enable him to put sufficient time and orderly thought into writing out carefully what was going on within him. (p. 317)

DATA COLLECTION

In explaining his phenomenal analysis, van Kaam (1983) used the example of the experience of really feeling understood to show how to begin an interview using his methods. He asked the participants to

> Describe how you feel when you feel that you are really being understood by somebody. (a) Recall some situation or situations when you felt you were being understood by somebody; for instance, by mother, father, priest, girlfriend (boyfriend), uncle, doctor, teacher, etc. (b) Try to describe how you felt in that situation (not the situation itself). (c) Try to describe your feelings just as they were. (d) Please do not stop until you feel that you have described your feelings as completely as possible. (p. 118)

DATA ANALYSIS

There are six operations in van Kaam's approach to analysis: listing and preliminary grouping, reduction, elimination, hypothetical identification, application, and final identification.

1. Classify data into categories. The researcher starts by taking a random sample of cases from the total sample of subjects' descriptions of the phenomenon being studied. The researcher then analyzes all the descriptive expressions found in the randomly selected samples and lists them. This beginning list is supplemented by other subjects' descriptions from the total sample in order to include every different descriptive description made by the subjects. A final listing needs to be agreed upon by expert judges. The researcher decides who the expert judges are. These chosen judges can have expertise in phenomenological research or expertise in the phenomenon under study.

2. The researcher reduces vague and overlapping descriptive expressions of the participants to more precise terms. At this step, intersubjective agreement with expert judges is required.

3. Any elements that are not describing the phenomenon being studied are eliminated.

4. Here the researcher composes the first hypothetical identification and description of the phenomenon being studied. It is termed hypothetical because at this point in data analysis, it is only a beginning draft.

5. The hypothetical description is applied to a randomly selected sample of cases. If there are a number of cases that do not correspond to the hypothetical description, then it is revised to match the evidence of the cases in the application. Next the operation of elimination of descriptions that do not pertain to the phenomenon is done. This revised hypothetical description is tested again with a new random sample of cases.

6. Once the above steps have been conducted successfully, then what was formerly known as the hypothetical identification of the phenomenon being studied is now considered to be a valid identification and description. The necessary and sufficient constituents of the phenomenon are synthesized into one description. Necessary constituents need to be in the majority of subjects' descriptions. van Kaam called for listing the constituents and then the percentages of subjects that expressed each one. In Table 5.1 is an example of this from his study of the feeling of being really understood.

The researcher justifies and explains each constituent element. First is a sentence that summarizes all of the constituents. Again, an example from the study on feeling understood is provided:

The experience of |"really | feeling understood"| is a perceptual-emotional Gestalt: | A subject, perceiving | that a person | coexperiences | what things mean to the subject | and accepts him, | feels, initially, relief from experiential loneliness, | and, gradually, safe experiential communion | with that person | and with that which the subject perceives this person to represent. (van Kaam, 1983, p. 120)

This statement is followed by the definition of each necessary constituent. Examples of his definitions for a couple of the constituents of the experience of really feeling understood are below:

Co-experiences: The understanding person shares at an emotional level the experiences of the subject understood. The prefix "co" represents the awareness of the subject that the person understanding still remains another.

Gradually, safe experiential communion: This expresses that the subject gradually experiences that the self is in the relieved, joyful condition of sharing its experience with the person understanding. "Safe" emphasizes that the subject does not feel threatened by the experience of sharing himself. (van Kaam, 1983, p. 121)

TABLE 5.1

Constituents of the Experience of "Really Feeling Understood"

Constituents of the Experience of "Really Feeling Understood"	Percentages Expressing the Constituents
Perceiving signs of understanding from a person	87
Perceiving that a person co-experiences what things mean to subject	91
Perceiving that the person accepts the subject	86
Feeling satisfaction	99
Feeling initially relief	93
Feeling initially relief from experiential loneliness	89
Feeling safe in the relationship with the person understanding	91
Feeling safe experiential communion with the person understanding	86
Feeling safe experiential communion with that which the person understanding is perceived to represent	64

EXAMPLES OF A STUDY FROM MY PROGRAM OF RESEARCH

I conducted a study of caring between nursing students and special needs children using van Kaam's methodology (Beck, 1992). The sample consisted of 36 nursing students who were asked to write about a caring experience they had with a special needs child during their pediatric rotation. Analysis revealed 199 descriptive experiences that resulted in six necessary constituents.

One expert judge reviewed the analysis for intersubjective agreement. The six necessary constituents and the percentages of nursing students expressing them are located in Table 5.2. Next I defined each constituent. Here are some of the definitions:

Authentic presencing: The nursing student puts all else aside and enters into the world of the child.

Physical connectedness: The nursing student and exceptional child embrace in touch. It can range from a gentle caress to an enthusiastic hug. This touching can be as tranquil as gently stroking a child's forehead and as exuberant and playful as tickling.

Reciprocal sharing: A meaningful interchange of selves occurs between the nursing student and exceptional child. This exchange involves feeling secure in a sharing of selves, of dreams for the future, and of time together.

Delightful merriment: The nursing student and the physically/mentally handicapped child are encompassed in happiness. Contagious smiles and laughter abound.

Unanticipated self-transformation: Unexpected changes emerge in the nursing student's attitude toward physically and mentally handicapped children. Unforgettable experiences with these exceptional children inspire the nursing student. (Beck, 1992, pp. 363–364)

The final step in analyzing the nursing students' descriptions was to synthesize these six constituents into one description: "A caring experience between

TABLE 5.2

Percentages of 36 Nursing Students Expressing Each Constituent

Constituents of Caring	%
Physical connectedness	92
Delightful merriment	83
Authentic presencing	80
Reciprocal sharing	75
Bolstered self-esteem	72
Unanticipated self-transformation	72

Source: Reprinted with permission from Beck, C. T. (1992b). Caring between nursing students and physically/mentally handicapped children: A phenomenological study. *Journal of Nursing Education, 31,* 361–366. p. 364.

a nursing student and an exceptional child is described as an interweaving of authentic presencing with physical connectedness and reciprocal sharing overflowing into delightful merriment, bolstered self-esteem, and an unanticipated self-transformation" (Beck, 1992, p. 363).

ADDITIONAL EXAMPLES OF STUDIES USING VAN KAAM'S DESCRIPTIVE PHENOMENOLOGICAL APPROACH

In Australia, Sumskis, Moxham, and Caputi (2017) used van Kaam's phenomenological approach to study the meaning of resilience in 14 schizophrenics. In Table 5.3 is an example of van Kaam's 4th step where the tentative relation of 11 structural elements are collated. Sumskis and colleagues also reported

TABLE 5.3
Elements Experienced as Being Supportive or Challenging

Elements (n=11)	Supportive	Challenging	Combination of Supportive and Challenging
Medication			X
Family			X
Work			X
Stimulation	X		
Stress		X	
Social ties			X
Stigma		X	
Lifestyle	X		
Physical health			X
Mental health system		X	
Mental health Professionals			X

Source: Reprinted with permission from Sumskis, et al. (2017). Meaning of resilience as described by people with schizophrenia. *International Journal of Mental Health Nursing, 26,* 273–284. p. 276.

the number of subjects out of the total sample of 14 who described the structural elements. For example, 11 participants described using medication and also maintaining a supportive family, and 10 participants described work in paid employment and managing stress. The 11 constituent elements were then synthesized to produce the following general structure of the meaning of resilience for schizophrenics:

> The meaning of resilience is embedded within an attitude of striving to overcome the severe adversity caused by schizophrenia. Striving enables the person to learn about themselves, the effect of schizophrenia on them, and how to manage schizophrenia in the context of the life they want to live. The process of striving involves struggle, and includes repeated, seemingly backward steps, while seeking out and utilizing supportive people and resources. The process of seeking out and using support also comes with challenges. Resilience is embedded within striving to competently overcome challenges in the quest for improvement. The person then uses resilience to seek out new challenges and experiences, and to grow life in ways unrelated to just living to manage schizophrenia. (Sumskis et al., 2017, p. 277)

A final illustration of van Kaam's methodology comes from a study on the experience of Recovery Camp in Australia for persons living with a mental illness (Picton, et al., 2018). Recovery Camp involved 5 days and 4 nights with university based students from a variety of disciplines at an adventure bush camp. There were specially designed programs to encourage the persons with a mental illness to extend themselves physically, socially, psychologically, and cognitively. Five of these campers participated in interviews asking them to describe what Recovery Camp was like for them. Picton et al. synthesized the meaning of empowerment in relation to the experience of Recovery Camp as "being determined to participate and extend oneself to strive physically, socially, and psychologically whilst being supported by positive relationships and leading to perceived positive changes" (Picton et al., 2018, p. 117).

CLARK MOUSTAKAS'S MODIFICATION OF VAN KAAM'S APPROACH

Clark Moustakas (1994) aligned himself with phenomenological research methods that are guided by the process of epoché, reduction, imaginative variation, and essences. Moustakas listed the following steps of his modification of van Kaam's approach:

1. List and do a preliminary grouping. Here every expression relevant to the experience under study is listed for each participant's description. Each expression has equal value. This is called horizontalization.

2. Determine the invariant constituents that are the unique qualities of the experiences that stand out. Does that expression contain a moment of the experience being studied that can be considered a necessary and sufficient constituent for understanding? Is it possible to abstract and label this expression? In this step, overlapping, vague, and repetitive expressions are deleted or expressed in more exact descriptive terms.

3. Cluster and thematize the invariant constituents. The researcher by means of imaginative variation and phenomenological reduction clusters the invariant constituents into core themes of the experience.

4. Final identification of the invariant constituents and themes by application: validation. In this step, the researcher checks the invariant constituents and their theme against the complete description provided by each participant. Here the researcher makes sure that (1) if they are expressed explicitly in the complete transcript, (2) if they are compatible if not explicitly expressed, and (3) if they are not explicit or compatible they should be deleted since they are not relevant to the participant's experience.

5. Individual textural description. From the thematic portrayals and validated invariant constituents, a textural description is constructed for each participant's experience.

6. Individual structural description. Each individual's structural description next is constructed based on their individual textural description and imaginative variation. A structural description includes a vivid portrayal of the underlying dynamics of the experience under study.

7. Individual-textural-structural description. A textural structural description of the constituent meanings and themes is developed for each participant.

8. Textural-structural synthesis. The final step involves developing a composite textural-structural description of the essence of the experience that represents the participants as a group. This description helps understand how the participants as a group experienced what they experienced.

EXAMPLES OF MOUSTAKAS'S MODIFICATION OF VAN KAAM'S APPROACH

The majority of current published studies using van Kaam's approach are based on Moustakas's (1994) modified approach. Researchers from various disciplines around the globe have used this modified methodology. For example, researchers from the discipline of Business examined the experience of decision makers in small businesses when considering expenditures for corporate social responsibilities (Dincer & Dincer, 2013). Another example from the discipline of Business focused on servant leadership in restaurant employee engagement (Carter & Baghurst, 2014). In Botswana, Mpuang, Mukhopadhyay, and Malatsi (2015) from the discipline of Education studied teachers' experiences of using sign language for learners who are deaf. Representing the Social Work discipline, Wright, Frost, and Turok (2016) explored the experiences of advanced practitioners with inserting a copper intrauterine device as emergency contraception. In India, Fargnoli (2017) from Creative Arts Therapies examined the experiences of self-care for human trafficking survivors.

From Information Technology, Alexander (2015) used Moustakas's modified van Kaam approach to explore 25 teachers' and counselors' perceptions of how to protect children from Internet predators. Five themes emerged: Lack of parental supervision, Social networking websites and chat rooms, Need for a relationship, Instant gratification, and Improved education. For each theme, Alexander specified the percentage of participant responses that cited the theme. For example regarding Theme 1, Lack of parental supervision, 12/40 or 30% of the participants cited this as the circumstance most likely to lead to teenagers' sexual encounters with a person they met on the Internet.

From the discipline of Curriculum and Instruction in Educational Leadership, Sullivan and Bhattacharya (2017) explored one retired teacher's experience of the evolution of the use of technology in the foreign language classroom. They used Moustakas's (1994) modification of van Kaam's approach. Four in-depth interviews were conducted with this educator over a period of 4 months as the retired teacher reflected on her 20 years of experience in the foreign language classroom. Each of Moustakas's essential steps was described with examples from this study. First Sullivan and Bhattacharya listed as codes all the expressions relevant to the experience from the interview transcripts. These were highlighted in yellow. Next in reduction and elimination, the researchers removed all the information not highlighted in yellow. In the following step a list of categories, known as invariant constituents, was made as the researchers combined similar categories in clusters of themes. The core themes were tested against the interview transcripts to determine the final identification of the invariant constituents.

TABLE 5.4

Sullivan and Bhattacharya's Sample of Coding and Clustering

What Teachers Did With Technology	What Students Do With Technology	Types of Technologies
Teacher could also communicate with each student individually cultural, just videos, cultural Cultural videos, but usually you had to check those out from a, like a media center Punch the right button or you were in trouble "Don't do it for me, show me how to do it so that I can learn"	Students listen to recordings Students could listen to recorded material and answer Obtain information Demonstrate comprehension Students watch and listen Complete written exercises based on the presentation Listening exercises I ask them for help when I get stuck They're always very nice and very good about showing me how to do things	Classroom that was equipped with headphones Headphones Cassettes Using a DVD program DVDs CDs Reel-to-reel Smart Boards Tape recorders Portable language labs Boombox iPad
Feelings	**Time Frames**	**Specifically Spanish**
Helpful in their own time Frustrating I'm glad I've had to use a computer in school I remember being very fearful A little scary I've learned not to be afraid Happy	Late 70s	Don't think we had programs for Spanish

Source: Reprinted with permission from Sullivan, N. B., & Bhattacharya, K. (2017). Twenty years of technology integration and foreign language teaching: A phenomenological reflective interview study. *The Qualitative Report, 22,* 757–778. p. 769.

Three major themes resulted: (1) Technology and different types available for teachers to use, (2) Technology integrated by the student and the educator, and (3) Looking to the future. In Table 5.4 is a portion of a table that Sullivan and Bhattacharya developed to provide a sample of their coding and clustering that helped the themes become concrete for them.

Sullivan and Bhattacharya (2017), following Moustakas's modification, then wrote an individual textual description, an individual structural description, and a textural-structural description that described the meanings and essences of the experience for the retired teacher incorporating the categories and themes. Here is an excerpt from the textural-structural description:

> 'I guess, you know, living in the moment and you don't think too far ahead as far as technology is concerned until it hits you over the head and you have to start using it (laughs)'. She wondered aloud about the direction of technology in the future and what was coming. She said that she 'often ask (her) students, what you think things are going to be like in 5 years, 10 years, when you have children of your own? What do you think they will be using?' (p. 768)

COMPARISON OF VAN KAAM'S METHODOLOGY AND MOUSTAKAS'S MODIFICATION

In data analysis, the first two steps of these methodologies are the same, namely, listing and preliminary grouping, and reduction and elimination. After that, however, the two methodologies definitely differ. At each step, van Kaam calls for intersubjective agreement with expert judges. Moustakas does not involve expert judges. Moustakas uses imaginative variation while van Kaam does not mention this in his methodology. It seems that van Kaam's methodology would require a larger sample than Moustakas's modification. In two of van Kaam's steps, the researcher selects a random sample of cases from the total sample while Moustakas does not include that at all. Moustakas's modification involves steps that are not part of van Kaam's methodology at all. These steps include constructing individual textural descriptions, individual structural descriptions, and individual textural-structural descriptions. The end product of Moustakas's modification is a composite description of the essence of the experience for the sample as a whole. van Kaam's end product consists of the necessary and sufficient constituents of the phenomenon synthesized into a succinct statement. Then this statement is followed by a definition of each necessary constituent.

In summary, this chapter focused on Adrian van Kaam's (1966) descriptive phenomenological methodology. Examples of studies conducted in the United States and Australia were presented. Also addressed in this chapter was Clark

Moustakas's modification. As a reminder, in Appendices A and B can be found the two student study guide activities. Next in Chapter 6, which follows, attention is now turned to the fourth descriptive phenomenological approach, that being, Dahlberg and colleagues' reflective lifeworld approach.

REFERENCES

Alexander, R. (2015). How to protect children from Internet predators: A phenomenological study. *Annual Review of Cybertherapy and Telemedicine.* doi: 10.3233/978-1-61499-595-1-82

Beck, C. T. (1992). Caring between nursing students and physically/mentally handicapped children: A phenomenological study. *Journal of Nursing Education, 31,* 361–366.

Carter, D., & Baghurst, T. (2014). The influence of servant leadership on restaurant employee engagement. *Journal of Business Ethics, 124,* 453–464.

Colaizzi, P. H. (1978). Psychological research as the phenomenologist views it. In R. S. Valle & M. King (Eds.), *Existential phenomenological alternatives for psychology* (pp. 48–71). New York, NY: Oxford University Press.

Dincer, B., & Dincer, C. (2013). Corporate social responsibility decisions: A dilemma for SME executives? *Social Responsibility Journal, 9,* 177–187.

Fargnoli, A. (2017). Maintaining stability in the face of adversity: Self-care practices of human trafficking survivor-trainers in India. *American Journal of Dance Therapy, 39,* 226–251.

Moustakas, C. (1994). *Phenomenological research methods.* Thousand Oaks, CA: SAGE.

Mpuang, K. D., Mukhopadhyay, S., & Malatsi, N. (2015). Sign language as medium of instruction in Botswana primary schools: Voices from the field. *Deafness and Education International, 17,* 132–143.

Picton, C., Patterson, C., Moxham, L., Taylor, E. K., Perlman, D., Brighton, R., & Hefferman, T. (2018). Empowerment: The experience of Recovery Camp for people living with a mental illness. *Collegian, 25,* 113–118.

Sullivan, N. B., & Bhattacharya, K. (2017). Twenty years of technology integration and foreign language teaching: A phenomenological reflective interview study. *The Qualitative Report, 22,* 757–778.

Sumskis, S., Moxham, L., & Caputi, P. (2017). Meaning of resilience as described by people with schizophrenia. *International Journal of Mental Health Nursing, 26,* 273–284.

van Kaam, A. (1966). *Existential foundations of psychology*. Pittsburgh, PA: Epiphany Association.

van Kaam, A. (1983). Phenomenal Analysis: Exemplified by a study of the experience of "really feeling understood." In A. Van Kaam (Ed.), *Foundations for personality study* (pp.117–123). Denville, NJ: Dimension Books.

van Kaam, A. (1987) *Scientific formulation: Formative spirituality* (Vol. 4). New York, NY: Crossroad Publishing Company.

Wright, R. L., Frost, C. J., & Turok, D. K. (2016). Experiences of advanced practitioners with inserting the copper intrauterine device as emergency contraception. *Women's Health Issues, 26*, 523–528.

Karin Dahlberg's Descriptive Phenomenological Reflective Lifeworld Research

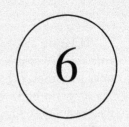

6

The focus of this chapter is first to introduce Dahlberg, Dahlberg, and Nyström's (2008) reflective lifeworld research. These researchers have developed two methodologies: One is for conducting a descriptive phenomenological study, and the second one is for a hermeneutic study. Chapter 6 concentrates on their descriptive phenomenological methodology. In Part III, which focuses on interpretive phenomenology, Dahlberg et al.'s hermeneutic methodology will be explained in Chapter 10.

....

INTRODUCTION TO THE REFLECTIVE LIFEWORLD METHODOLOGY

The reflective lifeworld research approach is based on the philosophies of Husserl (1970), Merleau-Ponty (1996), and Gadamer (2004). Dahlberg et al. (2008) developed their approach with common ground from phenomenology and hermeneutics. It is an open approach and not a method of a set of fixed rules. Reflective lifeworld researchers are viewed as being in "the flesh of the world" (Merleau-Ponty, 1968). As they participate in the relationship between themselves and the world, they experience and want to describe it. Openness and flexibility toward phenomena being studied are critical and require researchers to have a reflective attitude and not a natural attitude. Openness refers to the ability to be surprised and sensitive to the unpredicted and unexpected regarding what participants describe. Both phenomenology and hermeneutical traditions are concerned with researchers studying phenomena as they reveal themselves and not with imposing preconceived ideas on them. Lifeworld researchers must remain open to meaning as it is given.

Dahlberg and colleagues (2008) view phenomenological reduction as a critical initial step but felt this term was loaded with philosophical implications and instead chose the term "bridling." Openness is seen as the art of "bridling." In bridling, reflective lifeworld researchers focus on reflecting on their own lifeworld so that it does not go unnoticed in the research process. Bridling centers the researcher's energy to an open and respectful attitude that permits the phenomenon to present itself. Dahlberg and Dahlberg both live on horse ranches. They stress how researchers need to call on the same sensitivity and open attitude toward phenomena and their meaning as horse riders of the Spanish riding school, also known as academic horse riding. When these horse riders bridle their horses and make them dance, there is disciplined interaction and communication with their horses. Dahlberg et al. (2008) describe aspects of the attitude of bridling.

1. It involves researchers restraining their pre-understanding, which includes personal assumptions, beliefs, and theories.

2. It focuses on understanding the whole event and not just specific pre-understanding.

3. It points forward and not backward, as in bracketing, where the researcher's energy is focused on restraining pre-understanding.

In the reflective lifeworld approach, it is accepted that since researchers are part of the lifeworld, and in "the flesh of the world," it is not possible to bracket all pre-understanding, but it is possible to "bridle" understanding of the event with an awareness of our pre-understanding. Bridling characterizes the phenomenological attitude of scientific research that brings an attitude of carefulness and reflection. Dahlberg et al. (2008) emphasize that it is not a methodological technique but instead an art. A "bridled" researcher takes care not to make something definite when it is indefinite. The lifeworld is characterized by the natural, naïve attitude from which the world is understood. There is another attitude, one of reflection, in the lifeworld, which researchers need to practice. Through bridling, researchers are aware of their involvement in the world so that they can restrain their pre-understanding from preventing them from uncritically analyzing the data and forcing meanings to appear. In bridling, the researcher takes nothing for granted about the "real" existence of the phenomenon under study.

Research Question

The usual way a research question is written when using Dahlberg et al.'s approach is "What is the essence of the experience of . . .?"

Sample

Regarding sample size, Dahlberg and colleagues (2008) suggest researchers begin with about five interviews. Variation is more critical than the question of number. The aim of the reflective lifeworld approach is a general structure of a phenomenon that is dependent on each variation in the data. Data saturation is not a part of lifeworld research because meanings are viewed as infinite, always expanding so meaning saturation cannot exist.

Data Collection

Multiple data gathering methods can be used in the reflective lifeworld approach, such as interviews, biographies, observation, paintings, drawings, and fieldwork. Dahlberg et al. (2008) reminded researchers, as they engage with their participants and strive to maintain a direct and close relationship, that a reflective distance must also be kept, which they call the dance of lifeworld research. Dahlberg et al. (2008) explained that openness and ways to proceed for data gathering are essentially the same for descriptive phenomenological and hermeneutic research. Differences do appear, however, during data analysis. Descriptive phenomenological analysis aims at describing an essential structure of the phenomenon under study, while hermeneutic analysis involves interpretation; both are meaning oriented.

Lifeworld research is governed by the general principles of moving between the whole—the parts—the whole, which is central to understanding. As researchers analyze a text for meaning, they must address how each part is understood in regard to the whole and also how the whole is understood in regard to the parts. Gadamer (2004) called this the "hermeneutical rule." Others like the term "hermeneutic circle." Radnityky (1970) preferred to use the term "spiral" instead of circle to describe this process because the spiral is open at the beginning as well as at the end. Spiral is the term that Dahlberg et al. also prefer.

DESCRIPTIVE PHENOMENOLOGICAL REFLECTIVE LIFEWORLD APPROACH

Data Analysis

Now turning to Dahlberg et al.'s descriptive analysis in a phenomenological study, after dwelling with the transcribed text as a whole, attention is then focused on its different parts. Since researchers cannot analyze the entire text all at once, it is broken down into smaller segments called meaning units to help achieve a deeper understanding of the data. As an intermediate step on the way to a structure of meaning, researchers can make clusters of meaning. Dahlberg and colleagues noted that these clusters of meaning are not part of the results. These clusters just provide a temporary pattern of meanings to identify the essential meaning and structure of the phenomenon under study. Once the researcher is satisfied with the clusters of meaning, a return to the whole text is called for, now armed with a broader understanding than was initially thought. The clusters of meaning need to be related to each other to yield a pattern that describes the phenomenon as the researcher searches for its essence, its essential meanings, and its structure of meaning. The essence of a structure is that which makes a phenomenon what it is and without which it would no longer be that phenomenon. Dahlberg and colleagues (2008) described essences as being open, infinite, and expandable. Essences are never totally examined or described. To illuminate essence, researchers need to interrogate the data by asking questions to the text, such as, "What it says and how it is said. Does the text contain opposing statements? Does the participant express more than one understanding?"

Dahlberg et al. (2008) provide guidance for how the results of a descriptive phenomenological study should be presented. First the essence of the phenomenon is described. After that, the constituents that are the particulars of the structure are described. The essence needs to be seen in each constituent. By describing the constituents of a phenomenon, the researcher provides contextual aspects to the essence. The description of the essence in which the essential meanings of the phenomenon are described is written in the present tense. Dahlberg and colleagues call for the use of the present tense "because it describes how the phenomenon is, i.e., not what the informants said about it" (2008, p. 255). When presenting the essence, it should be written at a more abstract level than its constituents. Next, each constituent is described in-depth in order to emphasize all the subtle differences that were present in the data. Quotes from participants are added here. The complete description of the meaning structure includes general meanings along with individual lived meanings of the participants.

Dahlberg (2007) provides an example of her descriptive phenomenological reflective lifeworld research with her study of the phenomenon of loneliness. Her research questions guiding her study were "What is loneliness, What is its essence?" (p. 195). Dahlberg analyzed 26 interviews in order to describe the essential structure of this experience of loneliness. The following is an excerpt from the description of the essence of the experience of loneliness with its most invariant meanings.

> The phenomenon of loneliness stands out in meaning as "figure" against a "background" of fellowship with "important" people. In order to understand loneliness and its meanings, we must first consider this "background of fellowship" and its relation to loneliness. Fellowship with other people, to belong, appears in the interview material as fundamental to existence.

One can "be together with" other people, without them being particularly important in one's life. The absence of these particularly important people signifies the phenomenon of loneliness. One is lonely when these "important others" are not there, because one has either rejected them or they have "chosen to be rejected" and left the person behind, feeling lonely. . . . Loneliness as a phenomenon is characterized as transcending the immediate situation containing loneliness. One can feel lonely even if there are many people around, or one can be completely alone without feeling lonely. Loneliness can disappear with a sense of belonging, when one connects with someone who is miles away. (Dahlberg, 2007, p. 197)

Dahlberg then described the constituents of the meaning of loneliness, which included the following:

- Loneliness is to be without others

- Loneliness with others

- Loneliness is strange, wrong, ugly, or ever shameful

- Loneliness is restful and creative

- Companionship that constitutes the outer horizon of loneliness

Interdisciplinary Examples of Studies Using Dahlberg and Colleagues' Descriptive Phenomenological Approach

In this section, the following disciplines are represented: Geosciences and Natural Resource Management, Religious Studies, Occupational and Art Therapy, Nursing, Social Work, and Psychology. Petri and Berthelsen (2015) in Denmark described the essential meaning of everyday life experiences during curative radiotherapy in three patients with non-small-cell lung cancer (NSCLC). Using Dahlberg et al.'s (2008) reflective lifeworld approach, the researchers conducted a descriptive phenomenological study. Throughout their study, they practiced bridling where they took a critical reflective stance regarding their pre-understanding of the phenomenon under study. Below is an excerpt from the pre-understanding they bridled:

Patients with NSCLC receiving curative radiotherapy are not only struggling in an everyday life with symptoms and side effects of the treatment but also with feelings of guilt, shame, and stigmatization. We further believe that the needs of this patient group are overlooked in nursing as well as in the progress of standardized care and treatment. (p. 2)

Participants were interviewed in their homes and asked "how was a typical day for you during the radiotherapy treatment?" (Petri & Berthelsen, 2015, p. 3). Data analysis encompassed three phases: (1) reading and rereading the interview transcripts and dividing the text into meaning units, (2) grouping of meaning units into clusters, and (3) assembling the clusters of meaning in patterns. Table 6.1 is an illustration of these phases provided by Petri and Berthelsen for one constituent: A struggle for acceptance of an altered everyday life. The other three constituents of the essential meaning of the structure of this phenomenon included Radiotherapy as a life priority, Meeting the health care system, and

TABLE 6.1

The Three Phases of Dahlberg et al.'s Data Analysis Method Used by Petri & Berthelsen

1. Phase Reading and rereading of transcripts		2. Phase Grouping of meaning units into clusters	3. Phase Assembling the clusters of meaning in patterns
Excerpt from interview	Content	Meaning unit	Constituent
". . . my body said stop, I felt that . . . so I told myself that I could just do it tomorrow. . . ."	The side effects of the radiotherapy treatment are so disabling that the body says stop and the participant accepts that	Acceptance of a limited physical ability	A struggle for acceptance of an altered everyday life
". . . yes it has been tough, because I haven't had the energy to do anything else than radiotherapy. . . ."	The participant acknowledges that he only has energy to get the treatment		

Interpersonal relationships for better or worse. All four of these constituents were closely interrelated, and all were prerequisites of each other. Analysis revealed the essential meaning structure of everyday life during curative radiotherapy for patients with NSCLC as "characterized as hope for recovery serving as a compass through the changed everyday life" (p. 4).

In Norway from the discipline of Geosciences and Natural Resource Management, the lived experience of nature-based therapy in the University of Copenhagen's Nacadia Therapy Garden with persons suffering from stress-related illness was explored (Sidenius, Stigsdotter, Poulsen, & Bondas, 2017). Fourteen persons who were incapable of working due to stress-related symptoms participated in the 10-week, nature-based therapy. The participants were each interviewed three times using open-ended questions such as, "What is you impression of Nacadia?" Sidenius et al. (2017) used Dahlberg et al.'s (2008) descriptive phenomenological reflective lifeworld research approach. The researchers used bridling to maintain a critical reflective stance toward the phenomenon under study. Findings revealed that the essential meaning of nature-based therapy in Nacadia was captured by the phrase "I see my own forest and fields in a new way." Sidenius et al. (2017) identified and described the following seven constitutive elements:

> Another world of relationship and environments to habituate to; Becoming more comfortable and developing a sense of belonging; Suitable shelters offer less exposure and a sense of safety and freedom; Sensory experiences reinforced Nacadia as a supportive environment; Increased awareness of destructive mindsets; Spectrum of opportunities meeting individual capabilities and needs; and New approaches, more courage to change and move on. (p. 5)

Using a phenomenological reflective lifeworld research design, van Wijngaarden, Leget, and Goossensen (2015) from Religious Studies in the Netherlands explored the experience of 25 elderly people who felt their life was completed and no longer worth living. These researchers wanted to discover the essential characteristics of the phenomenon without which it would not be that phenomenon. Analysis revealed the essential meaning of "a tangle of inability and unwillingness to connect to one's actual life" (p. 260). The following five constituents were identified as components of the essential meaning of elderly persons feeling their life was completed and no longer worth living: (1) Sense of aching loneliness, (2) Pain of not mattering, (3) Inability to express oneself, (4) Multidimensional tiredness, and (5) Sense of aversion toward feared dependence.

In Sweden from Occupational and Art Therapy, Blomdahl, Wijik, Guregärd, and Rusner (2018) conducted a phenomenological reflective lifeworld research study and interviewed 10 persons diagnosed with moderate to severe depression about their experiences participating in a manual-based phenomenological art therapy. First the researchers described the essence of this phenomenon. Below is an excerpt from the essence:

> Manual-based phenomenological art therapy for people with moderate to severe depression means meeting oneself in an inner dialogue between the evident and the unaware. Art-making and the ensuing narrating makes inner life visible, and can open up and alter the understanding of oneself and one's situation. When an image is created, the image gives a visual response. The image acts as a mirror, which enables responding to the image by continuing to paint and develop the image. An interaction emerges between the participants, the material and the image. Through the image, and in the meeting and the interchange with oneself, an inner dialogue occurs. (Blomdahl et al., 2018, p. 20)

Next Blomdahl and colleagues presented the following four constituents of the essence:

- The inner dialogue takes place at various levels

- Overcoming challenges by perceiving and accepting oneself

- Frameworks enable the inner dialogues and the narrating of experiences

- Changes in understanding entail changes in life

From the discipline of Social Work in Israel, a descriptive phenomenological reflective lifeworld approach was used to investigate how aging persons with schizophrenia experience the self-etiology of their illness (Araten-Bergman, Avieli, Mushkin, & Band-Winterstein, 2016). Eighteen aging individuals with schizophrenia participated in in-depth interviews. Araten-Bergman et al.'s purpose was to describe the essence and meaning structure of the phenomenon under study. Meaning units or smaller parts of the transcripts were identified and clustered into patterns which led to a general structure that was the essence of the phenomenon and its constituents. Analysis revealed five constituents (pp. 1151–1152):

- "It leaves you to your fate" – schizophrenia as a decree of fate

- "I have sinned against God" – schizophrenia as a punishment from God

- "They put something in my coffee" – schizophrenia as a result of witchcraft

- "Her genes are in me" – schizophrenia as genetic

- "She left me and that's how I got sick" – schizophrenia as a result of personal trauma

Each of these constituents highlighted the interpretation of a different aspect of the phenomenon, and when put together made up / constituted the whole of the phenomenon.

Naidoo (2017) in South Africa from the discipline of Psychology used Dahlberg et al.'s (2008) phenomenological reflective lifeworld research approach to examine the daily lives of two children with cerebral palsy by means of interviews with the girls' teachers, mothers, and therapists. Naidoo described her process of bridling through her study so she could remain in an open and reflective attitude. She did peer checkings through discussions with an external auditor who was a child psychologist with qualitative research expertise. Naidoo strove to maintain a close relationship with her participants while keeping a reflective distance. Dahlberg and colleagues called this the dance of the lifeworld.

COMPARISON OF FIVE DESCRIPTIVE PHENOMENOLOGICAL METHODOLOGIES

Now that the descriptive phenomenological methodologies of these five phenomenologists have been explained, Table 6.2 summarizes a list of the data analysis steps of these methodologies. Four of the five methodologies come from Psychology and one from Nursing. Even though Colaizzi, Giorgi, and van Kaam's methods all come from the same Duquesne School of Phenomenology, differences are apparent among them (Beck, 1994). Colaizzi's (1978) approach is the only one that includes a final validation to be achieved by returning to the participants. van Kaam (1983) is the only one who calls for intersubjective agreement among expert judges at each step. While in Giorgi's (2009) and Dahlberg et al.'s (2008) methods, the outcome relies only on the researcher; they do not call for participant validation or the use of expert judges. Giorgi argued it is inappropriate for judges to be used. He went on to say "one does not need a judge as a half-way critic" (Giorgi, 1989, p. 77).

In data analysis, Colaizzi, van Kaam, and Moustakas eliminate repetitious statements, but Giorgi and Dahlberg et al. do not mention this. Giorgi keeps redundancies so the participant's entire description is kept. Colaizzi suggests that researchers can use their interrogated presuppositions about the phenomenon under study to assist in formulating research questions. van Kaam, on the other hand, claimed that researchers who start with their own analyzed

TABLE 6.2

Comparison of Five Descriptive Phenomenological Methods

Colaizzi	Giorgi	van Kaam	Moustakas	Dahlberg
Read all of the subjects' descriptions in order to acquire a feeling for them.	One reads the entire description in order to get a sense of the whole.	Listing and preliminary grouping of descriptive expressions that must be agreed upon by expert judges. Final listing presents percentages of these categories in that particular sample.	Listing & preliminary grouping.	Dwell with the transcribed text as a whole.
Return to each protocol and extract significant statements.	Researcher discriminates units from the participants' description of the phenomenon being studied. Researcher does this from within a psychological perspective and with a focus on the phenomenon under study. Giorgi states that each researcher does this from the perspective of his or her discipline. His method "is generic enough to be applied to any social science discipline."	In reduction the researcher reduces the concrete, vague, and overlapping expressions of the participants to more precisely descriptive terms. There again, intersubjective agreement among judges is necessary.	Reduction and elimination.	Text is broken down into smaller segments called meaning units.
Eliminate repetitious statements.			Clustering and thematizing invariant constituents.	
Spell out the meaning of each significant statement, known as formulating meanings.				
Organize the formulated meanings into clusters of themes.		Elimination of these elements that are not inherent in the phenomenon being studied or that represent a blending of this phenomenon with other phenomena that most frequently accompany it.	Final identification of invariant constituents and themes by application.	Make clusters of meaning as a temporary pattern.
Refer these clusters of themes back to the original protocols in order to validate them. At this point, discrepancies may be noted among and/or			Individual textural description.	Return to whole texts now with a broader understanding.

between the various clusters. Researchers must refuse temptation of ignoring data or themes which do not fit. Results so far are integrated into an exhaustive description of phenomenon under study. Formulate the exhaustive description of the investigated phenomenon in as unequivocal a statement of identification as possible. A final validating step can be achieved by returning to each subject asking about the findings so far.	Researcher transforms participant's natural attitude expressions into phenomenologically, psychologically sensitive expressions. Researcher synthesizes all of the transformed meaning units into a consistent statement regarding the participant's experiences called the structure of the experience. Researcher writes a specific structure for each participant and then a general structure.	A hypothetical identification and description of the phenomenon being studied is written. The hypothetical description is applied to randomly selected cases of the sample. If necessary, the hypothesized description is revised. This revised description must be tested again on a new random sample of cases. When operations described in previous steps have been carried out successfully, the formerly hypothetical identification of the phenomenon under study may be considered to be a valid identification and description.	Individual structural description Individual textural-structural description Individual textural-structural description of the group as a whole.	Relate clusters of meaning to each other to yield a pattern to help in search for the essence of the phenomenon. Illuminate the essence of the structure of the phenomenon. Identify the constituents that are the particulars of the structure that provide contextual aspects of the essence.

Source: Adapted from Beck, C. T. (1994). Reliability and validity issues in phenomenological research. *Western Journal of Nursing Research, 16,* 254–267.

experience may be prejudice from the very start. Dahlberg et al. (2008) views bridling as essential for researchers to reflect on their own lifeworld so it does not go unnoticed in the research process. When considering free imaginative variation, Dahlberg et al. and van Kaam do not mention this, but Colaizzi, Giorgi, and Moustakas do.

Knowing the ins and outs of each descriptive phenomenological methodology helps researchers choose which approach they will use in their study. For example, if researchers knew that they would not be able to return to their participants to provide feedback on the draft of their analysis, then Colaizzi's method would not be the best fit. If researchers knew they were going to have a large sample, then perhaps van Kaam's approach would be an appropriate choice. Researchers need to read the primary sources of those whose approach they choose to conduct their descriptive phenomenological study. Using primary sources to guide you in the design of your study is critical to conducting rigorous research and avoiding method slurring.

CHOOSING ONE OF THE DESCRIPTIVE PHENOMENOLOGICAL METHODS

Considering Colaizzi, Giorgi, van Kaam, Moustakas, and Dahlberg and colleagues' methodologies, why would you choose one over the other for a research study? One methodology is not better than the other. The choice depends on which one fits best with the research question and sample. For example, if you know that you can recruit a large sample, perhaps van Kaam's methodology would be a good fit since in order to use his approach you need a large enough sample to randomly select cases of the sample to apply the hypothetical description to. You also need a large enough sample to determine the percentages of each of the necessary constituents involved in van Kaam's approach. On the other hand, if you did not want to have expert judges check each of your steps, van Kaam's methodology would not be your choice.

Another aspect of a sample besides its size that can influence your choice of methodology is whether the researcher will be able to have access to the participants a second time to validate the tentative findings. Colaizzi calls his sample coresearchers and invites them to return to review the findings before a final structure of the experience is formed. If a researcher knows there is no possibility to be able to return to participants to validate results, Giorgi's approach may be a better fit since he says it is inappropriate for a researcher to ask participants to review the findings.

Dahlberg and colleagues' lifeworld research is an open design that is more flexible if this appeals to a researcher. They suggest multiple data gathering methods, such as paintings and observation, which can be attractive to some researchers. Dahlberg et al. explained that variation is more critical than the number of interviews. Data saturation is not the goal, in as much as meanings are viewed as infinite. They suggest beginning with five interviews. If a researcher foresees difficulty in obtaining a large sample size, maybe Dahlberg and colleagues' approach would fit nicely.

In summary, Dahlberg and colleagues' reflective lifeworld research method was introduced to set the stage for both their descriptive phenomenological methodology that was discussed in this chapter and also for their hermeneutic lifeworld research approach, to be covered in Chapter 10. Before moving on to the interpretive phenomenological methodologies that start in the next chapter, reasons why a researcher may choose one of the descriptive phenomenological methodologies over another are discussed. A reminder is that there are two student study activities located in Appendices A and B that faculty can assign their students to complete and share with their fellow classmates. Next, in Chapter 7 begins Part III of this book, where interpretive phenomenology takes center stage. Max van Manen's interpretive phenomenological approach is the focal point of this chapter that follows.

REFERENCES

Araten-Bergman, T., Avieli, H., Mushkin, P., & Band-Winterstein, T. (2016). How aging individuals with schizophrenia experience the self-etiology of their illness: A reflective lifeworld research approach. *Aging & Mental Health, 20,* 1147–1156.

Beck, C. T. (1994). Reliability and validity issues in phenomenological research. *Western Journal of Nursing Research, 16,* 254–267.

Blomdahl. C., Wijik, H., Guregärd, S., & Rusner, M. (2018). Meeting oneself in inner dialogue: A manual-based phenomenological art therapy as experienced by patients diagnosed with moderate to severe depression. *The Arts in Psychotherapy, 59,* 17–24.

Colaizzi, P. H. (1978). Psychological research as the phenomenologist views it. In R. S. Valle & M. King (Eds.), *Existential phenomenological alternatives for psychology* (pp. 48–71). New York, NY: Oxford University Press.

Dahlberg, K. (2007). The enigmatic phenomenon of loneliness. *International Journal of Qualitative Studies on Health and Well-Being, 2,* 195–207.

Dahlberg, K., Dahlberg, H., & Nyström, M. (2008). *Reflective lifeworld research.* Lund, Sweden: Studentlitteratur.

Gadamer, H.G. (2004). *Truth and method*. (2nd Revision). (J. Weinsheimer & D. G. Marshall, Trans.). London: Continuum.

Giorgi, A. (1989). Some theoretical and practical issues regarding the psychological phenomenological method. *Saybrook Review, 7*, 71–85.

Giorgi, A. (2009). *The descriptive phenomenological method in psychology: A modified Husserlian approach*. Pittsburgh, PA: Duquesne University Press.

Husserl E. (1970). *The crisis of European sciences and transcendental phenomenology* (D. Carr, Trans.). Evanston, IL: Northwestern University Press.

Merleau-Ponty, M. (1996). *Phenomenology of perception* (C. Smith, Trans.). New York, NY:Routledge.

Merleau-Ponty, M. (1968). *The visible and the invisible* (A. Lingis, Trans.). Evanston, IL: Northwestern University Press.

Naidoo, P. (2017). The negotiation of motor in/capabilities by two children with cerebral palsy as experienced by their carers. *The Indo-Pacific Journal of Phenomenology, 17* (Special edition: Positive Psychology), 12pp. doi: 10.1080/20797222.2017.1299288

Petri, S., & Berthelsen, C. B. (2015). Lived experiences of everyday life during curative radiotherapy in patients with non-small-cell lung cancer: A phenomenological study. *International Journal of Qualitative Studies on Health and Well-being, 10*: 29397. https://dx.doi.org/10.3402/qhw.v10.29397

Radnityky, G. (1970). *Contemporary schools of metascience*. Göteborg: Akademikerförlaget.

Sidenius, U., Stigsdotter, U. K., Poulsen, D. V., & Bondas, T. (2017). "I look at my own forest and fields in a different way": The lived experience of nature-based therapy in a therapy garden when suffering from stress-related illness. *International Journal of Qualitative Studies on Health and Well-being. 12*, 1324700. https://doi.org /10.1080/17482631.2017.132470

van Kaam, A. (1983). Phenomenal Analysis: Exemplified by a study of the experience of "really feeling understood." In A. Van Kaam (Ed.), *Foundations for personality study* (pp. 117–123). Denville, NJ: Dimension Books.

van Wijngaarden, E., Leget, C., & Goossensen, A. (2015). Ready to give up on life: The lived experience of elderly people who feel life is completed and no longer worth living. *Social Science & Medicine, 138*, 257–264.

PART III

Interpretive Phenomenology

Max van Manen's Hermeneutic Phenomenological Approach

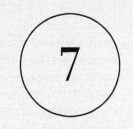

7

Max van Manen's (1990) hermeneutic phenomenological approach takes center stage in this chapter. He is a scholar from the Utrecht School of phenomenology in the Netherlands. The interplay of his six phases are explained. International examples of studies from the United States, Australia, Iran, India, and Denmark, where his methodology was used, are included to provide concrete examples of its application. These examples come from a variety of disciplines: Public Health, Pastoral Psychology, Nursing, Social Work, Physiology, Education, and Management.

Phenomenology is the science of examples (van Manen, 2017). Examples are methodologically a crucial part of phenomenological research. Through the singularity of an example of a phenomenon or experience researchers identify the exemplary aspects of the singular meaning of an experience. van Manen (2014) differentiated phenomenology from most other types of research. In phenomenology, the researcher studies the world as we ordinarily experience it or as we become conscious of it prior to our thinking or theorizing about it. The drive of phenomenological methodology is the wonder about how a phenomenon appears to us. The phenomenologist explains life as we live it; the lived experience. In this methodology, we investigate directly the prereflection dimensions of an experience. van Manen (2014) explained what he meant by his hermeneutic phenomenological method: "Hermeneutic means that reflecting an experience must aim for discursive language and sensitive interpretive devices that make phenomenological analysis, explication, and description possible and intelligible" (p. 26). He goes on to say that "ultimately, phenomenology is less a determinate code of inquiry than the inceptual search for meaning of prereflective experience" (p. 27). The aim of phenomenology is to grasp the essence of a phenomenon.

The epoché (bracketing) and reduction proper are two critical components of reduction. Reduction involves a continual questioning of how a phenomenon shows itself. The purpose of phenomenological research is to discover meaningful insights. van Manen (1990) reminded us that reduction is not simply a research method but a phenomenological attitude that needs to be adopted. The purpose of reduction is to gain access through the epoché to the prereflective experience in the world. If we are to understand the meaning of an experience, we need to reflect on it in order to be open and have an attitude of wonder. Reduction provides an attitude of wonder that only steps back far enough "to watch the forms of transcendence fly up like sparks from a fire; it slackens the intentional threads which attach us to the world and thus brings them to our notice" (Merleau-Ponty, 1962, p. xiii).

Hermeneutic reduction does not lead to a pure gaze, devoid of various preunderstandings. This is not possible. It leads instead to being continually open to questioning assumptions and preunderstanding. For van Manen (2014), bracketing a theory or body of knowledge on a topic does not mean to ignore it but instead to examine it for its possibilities "of extracting phenomenological sensibilities" (p. 226).

The use of the adjective "lived" with experiences indicates living through a prereflective or atheoretic experience. As van Manen (2017) explains:

> The instant of the moment we reflect on a lived experience, the living moment is already gone, and the best we can do is retrospectively try to recover the experience and then reflect on the originary sensibility or primordiality of what the experience was like in that elusive moment. (p. 812)

The challenge then for a phenomenologist is to recover lived meanings of a moment being careful not to objectify meanings as positivistic themes or objectified descriptions.

For van Manen (1990), hermeneutic phenomenological research consists of a dynamic interplay of six phases:

1. Turning to a phenomenon that seriously interests us and commits us to the world

2. Investigating experience as we live it rather than as we conceptualize it

3. Reflecting on the essential themes that characterize the phenomenon

4. Describing the phenomenon through the art of writing and rewriting

5. Maintaining a strong and oriented pedagogical relation to the phenomenon

6. Balancing the research context by considering parts and whole (pp. 30–31)

....

RESEARCH QUESTION

The purpose of phenomenology is to transform lived experience into a textual expression of its essence. As the researcher turns to the nature of lived experience, a phenomenological research question needs to be formulated. What is the nature of a particular lived experience? What is it like?

SAMPLE

Data saturation does not make sense for van Manen when doing phenomenology. He explained that in phenomenology understanding is "not a matter of filling up some kind of qualitative container until it is full or of excavating a data set of meaning until there is nothing left to excavate" (van Manen, Higgins, & van der Riet, 2016, p. 5). For van Manen, there is no saturation in regard to phenomenological understanding. Researchers cannot say they uncovered all the meaning of the phenomenon being studied. Therefore, he does not suggest a typical sample size.

DATA COLLECTION

Next, the researcher investigates the experience as it is lived. The researcher's personal experience is the starting point. Researchers explicate their assumptions and pre-understandings of the phenomenon. van Manen (1990) states that researchers being aware of their own experience of the phenomenon under study can perhaps provide researchers with cues to orient to the phenomenon. The researcher then obtains experiential descriptions of the phenomenon from others. van Manen offers a multitude of approaches for collecting other people's experiences: protocol writing, interviews, observation, experiential descriptions in literature, biographies, diaries, journals, and art as a source of lived experience. van Manen (1990) provided some suggestions for obtaining a lived experience description. When conducting an interview the participant is guided to do the following:

- Avoid generalizations or casual explanations.

- Describe the feelings, mood, and emotions that took place in the experience.

- Concentrate on a specific example of the experience.

- Focus on how the body felt, how things sounded or smelled during the experience.

- Avoid using fancy or flowery terms in the description.

Close observation is another way to collect experiential description. This involves participant observation. "Close observation involves an attitude of assuming a relation that is as close as possible, while retaining a hermeneutic alertness to situations, that allow us to constantly step back and reflect on the meaning of these situations" (van Manen, 1990, p. 69). When observing, the researcher writes anecdotes.

Researchers can also turn to poetry, literature, art, diaries, biographies, or personal life histories to increase practical insights to the phenomenon under study. In addition, researchers can use phenomenological literature that previously addressed the phenomenon. Another source includes the works of other phenomenologists. van Manen declared that using these selected phenomenological materials helps researchers to reflect in great depth on how we interpret this lived experience.

One of the best illustrations of van Manen's use of artistic sources to help bring themes to life is a study of mothers' experiences with the death of a wished-for baby (Lauterbach, 1993). In her inquiry into creative and artistic sources, Lauterbach used art, mourning painting, observation of memorial art in cemeteries, mourning photography, poetry, autobiography, historical literature, and music. Lauterbach found postmortem portraits of infants who had died during the 19th century America. She also discovered the depiction of her phenomenon in music. One example was a composition, "Kindertotenlieder" (Songs to Dead Children) written by Gustav Mahler in 1904.

DATA ANALYSIS

In the phase of hermeneutic phenomenological reflection, van Manen's approach helps researchers to grasp the essential meaning of the experience being studied. Here thematic analysis is conducted. Phenomenological themes "are more like knots in the webs of our experiences, around which certain lived experiences are spun and thus lived through as meaningful wholes" (1990, p. 90). Researchers can use three approaches to uncover themes: wholistic approach, selective approach, or a detailed approach. In a wholistic approach, the researcher tries to capture the meaning of the entire text. In the selective approach, the phenomenologist can highlight certain phases or statements that appear especially revealing about the experience. Lastly, in the detailed approach, every sentence is examined line by line. Once themes have been identified, researchers can go back to their participants in follow-up collaborative hermeneutic conversations when the participants reflect on deeper meaning of the themes. van Manen (1990) also suggests having collaborative hermeneutic conversations with a research seminar or group for the purpose of developing a more in-depth understanding of the phenomenon.

In reflecting on the essential meaning of an experience, there are four existential or fundamental lifeworld themes that van Manen (1990) suggested as being particularly helpful in the research process:

- Lived space (spatiality) which refers to filled space.

- Lived body (corporeality) focuses on the fact we are always bodily in the world.

- Lived time (temporality) refers to our subjective time not clock time.

- Lived human relation (relationality) is the relationship we maintain with other persons.

Once themes are identified, the researcher needs to call on free imaginative variation to help determine which themes are essential and which are incidental. An essential theme is one that makes the experience of phenomenon what it is and if taken away, then phenomenon would not be what it is.

For van Manen (1990), writing is not the last step in his research process. He argued that writing is a reflective part of his interpretive phenomenological method. Phenomenological writing does not just involve writing up the results. To write phenomenologically is to reflect. For van Manen, to write is to do research. More about writing a phenomenological study is addressed in Chapter 12.

EXAMPLES OF INTERNATIONAL RESEARCH FROM VARIOUS DISCIPLINES USING VAN MANEN'S METHODOLOGY

From Public Health, Waddell, Pulvirenti, and Lawn (2016) explored the experience of 20 female partners of male military veterans diagnosed with PTSD living in South Australia. The authors stated they used both detailed line by line analysis and the wholistic approach to reflect on the main themes. The researchers used van Manen's four phenomenological existentials of lived space, time, body, and human relations, to help analyze the data. Lived time referred not only to the temporal dimensions of past, present, and future but also to how time was perceived. In their theme of Lived human relation, the authors revealed how pervasive a partner with PTSD affected relationships with the veteran partner, relationships with others, and relationships with health care providers and the government.

In Pastoral Psychology, the lived experience of evangelical Christian pastors' counseling of members in their congregation who were victims/survivors of domestic violence was investigated in the United States (Zust, Housley, & Klatke, 2017). Using van Manen's interpretive phenomenology, the following five themes emerged: I'm not an expert on this, All I can do is spiritual, Anything to protect the children, It's not your fault!, and Solutions for a broken world. None of the pastors believed that they were adequately prepared to counsel their members regarding domestic violence. When children were in the family, the pastors concentrated on keeping the children safe and called child protective services. The message to the victims/survivors of domestic violence was that it was not their fault and the pastors reminded them how valuable they were to God.

From Social Work in the United States, Stensland and Sanders (2018) examined 21 older pain clinic patients' experiences living with chronic lower back pain. Guided by van Manen's approach, the main theme of "Living a life full of pain" emerged. Stensland and Sanders viewed the data through van Manen's four existential themes that encompass the lifeworld of humans: Lived space (spatiality), Lived body (corporeality), Lived time (temporality), and Lived self-other human relations (relationality). The participants' descriptions of their experiences living with lower back pain included four themes: (1) Corporeality: The pain is relentless and constantly monitored; (2) Temporality: To live with pain is to live by pacing day and night; (3) Relationality: Pain creates limits that can be tested or obeyed; and (4) Spatiality: Manipulating the space around me to accommodate the pain.

In Management, van Manen's approach was used by D'Cruz and Noronha (2018) in India to study the experience of workplace bullying on online labor markets. Thirteen Indian freelancers participated in telephone interviews to share their experiences of being targets of bullying, including racial harassment by clients and fellow freelancers. Interview transcripts were first analyzed using the sententious approach. Undergirding the participants' narratives was the core theme of "Pursuing long-term and holistic well-being", which touched on their resilience. Next using the selective approach, D'Cruz and Noronha examined the meaning of statements specifically in relation to the core theme and subthemes. Subthemes that dovetailed each other were combined into two major themes: Seeking resolution and Moving on.

Nurse researchers Larsen, Hall, Jacobsen, and Birkelund (2018) in Denmark explored the everyday life experiences of 14 women with systemic lupus erythematosus (SLE). Three consecutive interviews were conducted: the first one, then 6 months later, and finally 1 year later. Participants helped to interpret the data from their first two interviews in the third interview. van Manen's analytical steps of wholistic, selective, and detailed reading were completed. He suggested using artistic sources in helping to bring out the richness and fullness of themes. The researchers had an artist create a figure based on the metaphors and narratives of the participants' lives with SLE. The drawing was of moving waves with the participants portrayed as butterflies connected with the waves in a back and forth movement in life. Three themes were discovered: (1) Oscillating between the presence and absence of SLE, (2) Recognizing space and body possibilities and limitations, and (3) Being enriched through relationships and activities. van Manen (2014) suggested inviting participants to interpret pictures or poems. The drawing depicting the emerging themes was shared with the women during the third interview to assist with interpreting the results.

Groven, Råheim and Natvik (2017) from the discipline of Physiology used van Manen's method to explore the experiences of 10 Norwegian women as they practiced physical activity after weight loss surgery. During conversational interviews, the women were encouraged to elaborate on their experiences and to provide concrete, specific situations. The transcribed interviews were analyzed line by line to identify meanings, phrases, and metaphors. After the three researchers collaboratively interpreted the interview data, the following four themes emerged:

- Lived experiences of being physically active women

- Obligations and fear intertwined with fight against old eating habits

- Physical activity as risky

- Yoga as a means of being active despite fatigue and lack of energy

A phenomenological analysis of lifelong learning of vulnerable older adults was conducted in Canada using van Manen's approach (2014). From Education, Narushima, Liu, and Diestelkamp (2018) interviewed 10 participants between the ages of 70 to 90 about their experiences enrolled in general interest courses at a public continuing education program. These lower-income older adults continued to live independently in the community despite multiple risk conditions.

Following van Manen's suggestion, participants were asked to show the researchers artifacts that symbolized their learning. In their interpretive analysis, line by line readings and highlighting meaning units were done and then grouped into thematic clusters. Researchers searched for implicit meanings. Overarching themes and their subthemes were reclustered using the five existential aspects proposed by van Manen: Lived body, Lived time, Lived space, Lived relation, and Lived things. Narushima et al.'s major themes included the following:

- Assurance for the dissonant body and mind: Lived body (corporeality)

- A circle of camaraderie: Lived relation (relationality)

- A balance between physical and mental spaces: Lived space (spatiality)

- Integration of past, present, and future: Lived time (temporality)

- Beyond knowledge and skills: Lived things (materiality)

In summary, Max van Manen's interpretive phenomenological methodology was the focus of this chapter. Examples of international studies from various disciplines in which researchers used his approach were included. Students can be referred to the two student learning activities in Appendices A and B. In Chapter 8, Patricia Benner's interpretive phenomenology is highlighted. Her approach is the second of four types of interpretive phenomenology addressed in this book.

REFERENCES

D'Cruz, P., & Noronha, E. (2018). Target experiences of workplace violence bullying on online labour markets: Uncovering the nuances of resilience. *Employee Relations, 40*, 139–154.

Groven, K. S., Råheim, M., & Natvik, E. (2017). Practicing physical activity following weight loss surgery: The significance of joy, satisfaction, and well-being. *Indo-Pacific Journal of Phenomenology, 17*(2), 10.1080/20797222.2017.1370903

Larsen, J. L., Hall, E. O. C., Jacobsen, S., & Birkelund, R. (2018). The existential experience of everyday life with systemic lupus erythematosus. *Journal of Advanced Nursing, 74*, 1170–1179.

Lauterbach, S. S. (1993). In another world: A phenomenological perspective and discovery of meaning in mothers' experience with the death of a wished-for baby: Doing phenomenology. In P. Munhall & C. Oiler (Eds.), *Nursing research: A qualitative perspective* (pp. 133–179). New York, NY: National League for Nursing Press.

Merleau-Ponty, M. (1962). *Phenomenology of perception*. London: Routledge and Kegan Paul.

Narushima, M., Liu, J., & Diestelkamp, N. (2018). I learn, therefore I am: A phenomenological analysis of meanings of lifelong learning for vulnerable older adults. *The Gerontologist, 58*, 696–705.

Stensland, M., & Sanders, S. (2018). Living a life full of pain: Older pain clinic patients' experience of living with chronic low back pain. *Qualitative Health Research, 28*, 1434–1448.

van Manen, M. (1990). *Researching lived experience*. London, Ontario, Canada: The State University of New York.

van Manen, M. (2014). *Phenomenology of practice*. Walnut Creek, CA: Left Coast Press, Inc.

van Manen, M. (2017). Phenomenology in its original sense. *Qualitative Health Research, 27*, 810–825.

van Manen, M., Higgins, I., & van der Riet, P. (2016). A conversation with Max van Manen on phenomenology in its original sense. *Nursing and Health Sciences, 18*, 4–7.

Waddell, E., Pulvirenti, M., & Lawn, S. (2016). The lived experience of caring for an Australian military veteran with Posttraumatic Stress Disorder. *Qualitative Health Research, 26*, 1603–1613.

Zust, B. L., Housley, J., & Klatke, A. (2017). Evangelical Christian pastors' lived experience of counseling victims/survivors of domestic violence. *Pastoral Psychology, 66*, 675–687.

Patricia Benner's Interpretive Phenomenological Methodology

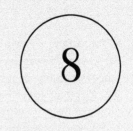

8

Patricia Benner's (1994) interpretive phenomenological approach is addressed in this chapter. The use of her three interrelated interpretive strategies of identifying paradigm cases, exemplars, and thematic analysis are described. Studies conducted in the United States, Sweden, Nigeria, and Italy are presented to illustrate the use of her methodology. Researchers from various disciplines employed her approach, such as Education, Law, and Nursing.

For Benner, a Heideggerian phenomenology is a systematic approach to interpreting the transcribed text of interview material and observations. Her phenomenology leads to explanation and prediction that yields understanding and choice, not manipulation and control. Interpretation proceeds from analysis of the whole text, to parts of the text, and a comparison of these interpretations. In the hermeneutic circle, there is a shifting back and forth between the parts and the whole. Here the researcher enters into a dialogue with the text to search for commonalities in meanings.

The researcher's own background knowledge is part of the perceptual lens for conducting a study. Researchers undergo critical reflective exercises of their biases and assumptions to create a sense of openness so they are able to hear questions they might not have considered prior to analyzing the texts. As researchers make explicit their assumptions at the start of a study, these should be considered tentative, and researchers need to permit their assumptions to be challenged and transformed through interpreting the participants' voices. The researcher's interpretive analysis involves clarifying distinctions and similarities across cases to identify general categories or general themes. Researchers seek to provide greater understanding to the texts for the reader by providing meanings and qualitative distinctions. In interpreting the text, researchers ask, "What do I now know or see that I did not expect or understand before I began reading the text?" (Benner, 1994, p. 101). She warned that if researchers' own views have not been challenged or broadened, the quality of the research can be questioned due to the danger of the researchers just relying on their preconceptions. For Benner, understanding must be understood historically. Researchers need to keep track of their steps in understanding. For instance,

> "When I understood the text from this aspect, I saw these issues and themes, but when I began to consider conflicting stories and events and to hear certain arguments within the text, I was able to see new issues and new clearings." (Benner, 1994, p. 101)

SAMPLE

Benner (1994) explained that sample size is determined by the size of the text. At the start of a study, a researcher estimates the sample size, but this number is adjusted many times based on the quality of the texts. Projected sample size should take into account repeated interviews and/or observations with the participants. The larger the total text, the more opportunity it allows for redundancy and clarification and an adequate range of situations.

DATA COLLECTION

When interviewing participants, Benner (1994) stressed the importance of conducting interviews in a naturalistic way, avoiding abstract language, academic, or research terms. Use of more conversational everyday language helps the participants feel more comfortable in order to share their experiences and feelings in their ordinary pattern. In interpretive phenomenology, storytelling is key because it allows participants to describe their own narratives about their experience and not just provide facts and opinions. It is important for the researcher to listen and not interrupt the participant's storytelling. Language that is imaginative and pictorial is helpful in interviewing. Benner (1994) provided some examples of this: "How would you think that looked to others? Do you think anyone else would have known how you were feeling?" (p. 111). When researchers introduce practical contrasts, this encourages participants to provide a fuller, richer account of their personal experiences. In interpretive phenomenology, researchers need to confirm what they understood in the participant's narrative. Open listening helps the researchers know they have understood what the participant had shared. In open listening, the researchers allow participants to shape the telling of their story that leads to obtaining a broader contextual narrative of participants' experience.

After open listening, the researchers can follow up with the participant to make sure that they understood what the participant said. This type of listening is called active listening. In active listening, researchers paraphrase their understanding of what the person said. For Benner (1994), the interpretive dialogue starts with the first interview. Collecting data and analyzing data are not separated. This permits researchers to follow up on questions that emerge from the study itself.

The multiple stages of interpretation permit some bias control by helping expose contradictions or surprises. Benner (1994) warned that researchers interpreting the voices of their participants can never escape their taken-for-granted background that leads to the possibility of an interpretive foreground. Benner is a strong proponent of multiple interviews with the same participants as another bias control strategy. Multiple interviews help the researcher to see emerging patterns and prevent emphasizing an action, statement, or episode that is non-recurring. The more redundant findings are, the more confidence one can have in the interpretation. Multiple interviews give researchers the opportunity to review the audiotape before the next interview. This permits the researcher and participants a second chance to ensure that understanding occurred.

Data collection can include a variety of sources, such as participant observation, videotapes, documents, media, and photographs, to name a few. Also, photographs and videotapes can disclose aspects of a situation that may be unnoticed by the researcher. Allowing participants to take their own photographs of their experience can have the advantage of being privy to their emotions and concerns that may not be present in an interview.

In addition to individual one-on-one interviews, small-group interviews are an effective data collection approach. Benner (1994) explained the purposes of small group interviews:

- Allows peers to converse with one another for telling their stories

- Permits active listening as multiple listeners are trying to understand another person's story

- Enriches the meaning of stories as they trigger similarities and differences among different persons' narratives

DATA ANALYSIS

Benner (1985) suggested three interrelated strategies to permit particular claims of the text to stand out: paradigm cases, exemplars, and thematic analysis. These interpretive strategies work for both discovery and presentation strategies. Benner called a paradigm case a marker that is a whole case that portrays a strong example of a specific pattern of meanings. Paradigm cases are usually the entering point of analysis. This marker brings clarity and vividness and helps identify other cases with similar characteristics that are more subtle. Early in interpreting, paradigm cases are especially helpful because the researcher may recognize the case as a strong example of a specific meaning or relationship but cannot at this early stage understand why the case stands out or what it is pointing out. The researcher systematically moves back and forth from parts of the text to the whole text to check for incongruities, concerns, and puzzling aspects. By comparing this case to other cases, the researcher can identify what the paradigm case is depicting. Once the first paradigm case is constructed, the researcher examines a second case in regard to the first paradigm case. Comparison of similarities and differences among paradigm cases is looked for. Use of paradigm cases allows the reader to engage in the practical world of the participants and to be closer to their experience.

An exemplar is smaller than a paradigm case but can also provide strong examples of a specific meaningful transaction that helps others identify similar meaningful transactions in different situations where the characteristics may be very different. The interpretive process focuses on the analysis of specific episodes or incidents. Exemplars illustrate aspects of a paradigm case or a thematic analysis. Benner suggests that keeping track of exemplars the researchers have chosen as illustrative of a pattern allows them to follow their train of thought. Collection of exemplars is viewed by Benner (1994) as central to the interpretive task. A range of exemplars helps establish the relationships and distinctions the researcher is making.

An example of a paradigm case is one Wros (1994) presented in her study of nursing care of dying patients in critical care. She entitled the paradigm "do no harm", which described nurses' caring for a young woman dying of complications of cancer treatment. Wros added supportive exemplars, specific to this case, to further illustrate and enhance the understanding of this paradigm case.

Thematic analysis is Benner's (1985) third interpretive strategy. In thematic analysis, the researcher moves back and forth between sections of the text and segments of the analysis to clarify distinctions and similarities across cases. Shifting can be from themes and situations and from thematic analyses to paradigm cases. Meaningful patterns are identified rather than small units like words or phrases. Benner (1994) explained that this shifting between parts and whole of a text permits the researcher to develop additional interpretive questions. The researcher is involved in cycles of understanding, interpretation, and critiques. Here common themes are identified from the interviews. Excerpts from the interviews should be included to provide evidence for the readers of the themes. Benner argued that with all three analytic and presentation strategies, the researcher needs to present enough documentation from the interviews so that readers will be able to validate the findings.

In her approach, Benner (1985) argued for expert consensual validation for at least a subset of the data to make certain the meanings are supported by the text. One of her underlying assumptions in her method is that interpretations that are offered have their basis in shared cultural meanings and consequently should be recognized by other readers from the same culture. Review by other researchers can help alert the researcher uncover blind spots and questions that were avoided in interviewing. Benner called for respect for commonalities and differences between the researcher and participants. This is accomplished by dialogue and listening that permits the voices of the participants to be heard.

Interpretive phenomenologists are interested in commonalities, and Benner and Wrubel (1989) identified five sources of commonality explored in phenomenology: situation, embodiment, temporality, concerns, and common meaning.

- Situation: Here the researcher concentrates on understanding how the participant is situated historically and presently.

- Embodiment: An understanding of embodied knowing includes perceptual, bodily, and emotional responses.

- Temporality: The lived experience of time is the focus here as the researcher understands how the participants project themselves into the future but also understands oneself from the past.

- Concerns: These are what matter to the participants.

- Common meanings: These refer to taken-for-granted meanings that form what is noticed and what the issues are between persons.

Brykczynski and Benner (2010) stated that there is no stepwise formula that researchers can use in conducting an interpretive phenomenological study; however, there are some practices that are typical of this approach:

- Use of participant observations and interviews for data collecting

- Use of interviews to capture the temporal progression of situations in each participant's narratives

- Use of three interrelated interpretive strategies for identifying paradigm cases, exemplars, and thematic analysis

- Use of a research team for interpreting the data

INTERNATIONAL EXAMPLES OF STUDIES USING BENNER'S INTERPRETIVE PHENOMENOLOGICAL METHODOLOGY

In Sweden from the Department of Clinical Science and Education, Mattisson, Arman, Castren, and Forsner (2014) examined the meaning of caring in a pediatric intensive care unit (PICU) from the perspective of parents. Interviews and observation were conducted with 11 parents of seven children. Reflection, interpretation, and the use of the hermeneutic circle were all employed by the researchers. The observations ranged from 2 to 4 hours of bedside caring situational observations in order to capture the situatedness of the interaction with children and their parents. Follow-up interviews were conducted in the PICU with parents to explore their experiences of how their child was cared for in the PICU focusing on pain management and caring. During data analysis, the researchers switched back and forth between the whole and the parts of the interview texts in order to gain the meaning. Mattsson and colleagues used a four-phase process described by Brycznski and Benner (2010): (1) data collection as well as verbatim transcription of interviews and observation notes, (2) interpretation of exemplars, (3) sentences that reflected the parents' experiences were compared, and (4) themes and subthemes were identified. When interpreting the exemplars, the researchers kept three questions in mind:

- Is this what the meaning of caring really is?

- Is this an experience of caring and how does caring show up in this example?

- If we leave this out, would it alter our understanding of the meaning of caring? (Mattsson et al., 2014, p. 340)

Four themes emerged that together revealed the significant meaning of parents' perspective of caring in the PICU: (1) Being a bridge to the child on the edge, (2) Building a sheltered atmosphere, (3) Meeting the child's needs, and (4) Adapting the environment for family life. Mattsson et al. (2014) included the following excerpt to show how "bridging" opened up possibilities that nurses helped the parents to meet their child's needs and reconnect with them in the illness:

> They talked a lot, like, now we are going to put a tube in your throat. Now, I'll touch your right hand a bit, and will hold here so now we are going to, now you'll feel a bit cold here. When I sat beside and felt, wow, he understands me, I can also talk like that to him. After that I talked more with him, read more, talked to him. (p. 341)

In the discipline of Law, Benner's (1994) interpretive phenomenology was used by Usman, Yaacob, and Rahman (2015) to explore the challenges of consumer protection in the Nigerian deregulated sector. The researchers chose Benner's approach because they said it emphasized studying the everyday experiences and knowledge of the challenges of consumer protection. Twenty participants who were staff from consumer protection and products standard-setting agencies, heads of consumer organizations, and academics were interviewed. Benner's thematic analytical approach guided the main theme of lack of awareness as the major challenge for consumer protection. Subthemes included Lack of consumer education, Ignorance of the consumers, and Lack of consumers' knowledge regarding their rights, redress avenues, and consumer protection laws. Usman et al. hoped their findings would help their government draw up policies and measures to improve electricity consumers' welfare in Nigeria.

Posttraumatic stress experiences of 67 wounded male servicemen in the Afghan and Iraq wars plus 401 nurses' experiences providing care for solders injured in these wars were investigated (Benner, Halpern, Gordon, Popell, & Kelley, 2018). These researchers primarily conducted small-group interviews consisting of two to six persons. The wounded male servicemen and the nurses were interviewed separately. Using Benner's interpretive phenomenological approach, powerful paradigm cases of the nurses and servicemen were developed, such as one of a soldier being blown up in the air from an improvised explosive device (IED) while walking. This paradigm case helped illustrate the theme of Lifeworld: The powerful, formative experience of being "there" and "then." Here is an excerpt from this paradigm case:

> While walking, the IED just dropped out of nowhere. I thought a mortar landed on us, because I felt the debris rush through my body. But at the same time. I closed my eyes, but I remember feeling everything—I was doing back flips, cartwheels. But I remember floating in the air. When I opened my eyes, I was at least 50 meters from where I was walking. . . . I felt kind of dazed and confused, but I thought something had happened, but I didn't determine how bad it was. I tried to get back up, I couldn't. I tried to pick up the equipment but it was made into pieces, nothing. I just found myself looking up in the sky. It was very blue and—I don't know, it was just a beautiful day but . . . I was laughing. "If I was to die today it would be a beautiful today to die." (Benner et al., 2018, p. 51)

An example of a theme related to the nurse veterans was entitled Not being able to be here: Acute grief, general anxiety, inability to focus. Nurses' generalized anxiety left over from the dangerous war zone and their detachment as a coping mechanism hindered these nurses from being fully present with their military patients. Some of the other themes included Embodied responses to environmental cues "here" as if they were "there"; Being "here" while longing to be "there"; and Stigma, social isolation, and detachment "here" after being "there."

In Italy, Tolotti et al. (2018) used Benner's interpretive phenomenology to investigate the communication experience of tracheostomy patients with nurses in the intensive care unit (ICU). From the discipline of Nursing, their research question was, "What is the lived experience of adult patients with a tracheostomy, who are not under sedation and mechanically ventilated, in their communication with nurses during their stay in the ICU?" (p. 25). The researchers collected data in three ways: participant observation while patients were in the ICU, in-depth interviews with eight patients after they left the ICU, and situated interviews with the seven nurses whom the patients remembered best in their communication experiences. Benner encouraged the use of participant observation as another valuable way to collect data. These observations were conducted while the patients were still in the ICU. The researchers shared a list of observation items they focused on. Examples of these items included conditions of the tracheostomy patient (posture, presence of infusions, level of sedation); care activities each nurse provided to each patient; and nonverbal communication of both patients and nurses. Tolotti et al. (2018) conducted between three and five observations with each patient.

First in data analysis, Tolotti et al. (2018) did a line-by-line thematic analysis of the eight patients' interview transcripts. The primary themes were identified and put into categories, reflecting on their potential meanings. Next, themes were identified from the seven nurses' transcripts. For each case, Tolotti and the rest of her team noted similarities and differences between the patients' and nurses' transcripts. Focus was placed on the communication difficulties patients experienced and the comfort and discomfort factors involved in communicating with nurses. Two themes emerged regarding communication experiences with nurses: (1) Feeling powerless and frustrated due to the impossibility of using voice to communicate and (2) Facing continual misunderstanding, resignation, and anger during moments of difficulty and/or communication misunderstandings. Similarities and differences in the themes when comparing patients' and nurses' experiences were highlighted. Interwoven throughout the findings were excerpts from the interviews to provide evidence for the readers regarding the identified themes.

In summary, the interpretive phenomenology of Patricia Benner was covered in this chapter along with supportive examples of studies from around the globe. In Appendices A and B are located two student study activities.

Next, in Chapter 9, the third of four methodologies for conducting interpretive phenomenology is the focus. This method is that of Smith and colleagues' interpretive phenomenological analysis.

REFERENCES

Benner, P. (1985). Quality of Life: A phenomenological perspective on explanation, prediction, and understanding in nursing science. *Advances in Nursing Science, 8*, 1–14.

Benner, P. (Ed.) (1994). *Interpretive phenomenology: Embodiment, caring, and ethics in health and illness.* Thousand Oaks, CA: SAGE.

Benner, P., Halpern, J., Gordo, D. R., Popell, C. L., & Kelley, P. W. (2018). Beyond pathologizing harm: Understanding PTSD in the context of war experience. *Journal of Medical Humanities, 39,* 45–72.

Benner, P. & Wrubel, J. (1989). *The primacy of caring: Stress and coping in health and illness.* Reading, MA: Addison-Wesley.

Brykczynski, K. A., & Benner, P. (2010). The living tradition of interpretive phenomenology. In G. Chan, K. Brykczynski, R. Malone, & P. Benner (Eds.), *Interpretive phenomenology in health care research* (pp. 113–141). Indianapolis, IN: Sigma Theta Tau International.

Mattsson, J. Y., Arman, M., Castren, M., & Forsner, M. (2014). Meaning of caring in pediatric intensive care unit for the perspective of parents: A qualitative study. *Journal of Child Healthcare, 18,* 336–345.

Tolotti, A., Bagnasco, A., Catania, G., Aleo, G., Pagnucci, N., Cadorin, L. . . . Sasso, L. (2018). The communication experience of tracheostomy patients with nurses in the intensive care unit: A phenomenological study. *Intensive and Critical Care Nursing, 46,* 24–31.

Usman, D. J., Yaacob, N., & Rahman, A. A. (2015). Lack of consumer awareness: A major challenge for electricity consumer protection in Nigeria. *Asian Social Sciences, 11,* 240–251.

Wros, P. L. (1994). The ethical context of nursing care of dying patients in critical care. In P. Benner (Ed.), *Interpretive phenomenology: Embodiment, caring and ethics in health and illness* (pp. 255–277). Thousand Oaks, CA: SAGE.

Jonathan Smith's Interpretive Phenomenological Analysis

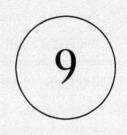

Jonathan Smith, Paul Flowers, and Michael Larkin's (2009) interpretive phenomenological analysis (IPA) is the focal point of this chapter. The six steps in their method are described along with research examples from the disciplines of Clinical Speech and Language, Human Movement Sciences, Music Therapy, Family Therapy, and Medicine. These studies were conducted in Ireland, UK, Canada, Australia, and the United States.

Interpretive phenomenological analysis (IPA) comes from the discipline of Psychology (Smith et al., 2009). Smith (1996) labeled his method interpretive phenomenological analysis for the dual nature of its approach. One approach was to explore participants' experiences of the world and provide an insider's view. The second approach was that this access to participants' experiences is complicated by the researcher's own conceptions, which are needed to make sense of the participants' world through interpretation. Key principles that are at the heart of this approach include the following: (1) the research is focused on exploring "the thing itself" (p. 186), which is the phenomenological experience of the participant, (2) researchers have an intense interpretative engagement with the description provided by the participant, and (3) each participant's description of the experience is examined in detail. IPA has three main theoretical underpinnings: phenomenology, hermeneutics, and ideography (Smith, 2017). Ideography refers to being concerned with the particulars and focusing on the meaning of something for a given person. It involves detailed examination of a particular experience for a person.

RESEARCH QUESTIONS

Since IPA is concerned with a detailed investigation of experience, Smith et al. (2009) suggested that a research question should not be on too grand a scale. Primary research questions should be focused on participants' understanding of their experiences. Research questions are open and directed toward meaning.

In Smith et al.'s method, researchers can also have secondary- or theory-driven research questions. These types of questions can be answered only in the interpretative stage of analysis. Secondary research questions engage with a theory but do not test it.

SAMPLE

Samples are obtained purposively and often by means of referrals from gatekeepers or by snowballing where your participants make referrals. One criterion is that an individual represents a perspective on the phenomenon being studied rather than a population. Small sample sizes are typical in IPA studies. The detailed case-by-case analysis of each participants' interview transcripts is time consuming. Smith and colleagues suggest that IPA researchers recruit a homogeneous sample. If groups are more homogeneous, a researcher can investigate in detail the variability within that group. Convergence and divergence within the group can be analyzed. Regarding sample size, Smith et al. (2009) explained that there is no correct answer. Sample size will depend on such factors as how rich the data from individual cases are and organizational constraints the researcher is working under. Single-case studies are a possibility in the IPA method. A reasonable sample size for a student's project is between three and six participants.

DATA COLLECTION

In-depth interviews are a staple in IPA studies. These interviews can be semistructured or unstructured. Smith et al. (2009) suggested researchers new to qualitative methods develop a semistructured interview that consists of between six to 10 open-ended questions for adults. Here is a suggested sequence for developing a semistructured interview schedule:

1. Decide on the broad area which you want your participants to discuss.

2. Consider the range of topic areas that you want your interview to address.

3. Arrange the topics in the most appropriate sequence. For example, sensitive issues need to be gradually worked toward.

4. Decide on what phrases you will use to open questions focusing on each broad area.

5. Have others review your tentative list of questions. A potential participant or another researcher are appropriate choices.

More experienced qualitative researchers may choose to use unstructured interviews. With this type of interview, there is usually one core interview question to begin the interview. Then how the interview develops will depend completely on how the participant responds to that first opening question. Sometimes IPA researchers may find it useful to collect additional data that can assist in contextualizing the interview transcript, such as participant observation.

Smith and colleagues identified what they called bolder designs. One option in a bolder design is to interview each participant multiple times, and another option is a longitudinal design. Exploring a phenomenon in multiperspectival studies is yet another bolder design where the researcher explores the phenomenon from multiple perspectives.

DATA ANALYSIS

Smith et al. (2009) developed six steps in their IPA for analyzing the descriptions provided by the participants' interviews.

Step 1. Reading and rereading

Here the researchers immerse themselves in the data, reading and reading again the transcripts from the participants' interviews.

Step 2. Initial noting

Smith et al. (2009) stated that this is the most detailed and time-consuming feature of the analysis. Researchers start to write notes on the transcripts. Three types of comments can be made. Descriptive comments focus on the content of what the participant shared regarding the phenomenon being studied. Linguistic comments specifically explore the participant's use of language. Conceptual comments concentrate on the researcher's engagement at a more interpretive and conceptual level. In this step, Smith and colleagues suggest using decontextualization to help lead to a detailed focus on the participant's words and meanings. One strategy for achieving this is to take apart the narrative flow of the transcript by taking one paragraph at a time and reading it backward to obtain a feel for the use of specific words.

Step 3. Developing emergent themes

Here the researchers analyze their exploratory comments to determine emergent themes. Focus is on specific chunks of the transcripts. The whole of the narrative is fragmented to reorganize the data. In changing exploratory comments into themes, researchers concentrate on writing a concise statement regarding what was important in that note. Phrases can be used that include the psychological essence of that comment. In the hermeneutic circle, the part is interpreted in relation to the whole, and the whole is interpreted in relation to the part.

Step 4. Searching for connections across emergent themes

At the start of this step, researchers have a set of emergent themes within each transcript. These emergent themes are ordered in how they present in the transcripts. Now the challenge for the researchers is to look for connections between the themes in each transcript to fit the themes together. Smith et al. (2009) suggested six ways researchers can look for patterns and connections among emergent themes.

- Abstraction involves clustering like with like in a "superordinate" theme and giving it a new name.

- Subsumption occurs when an emergent theme itself is considered a superordinate theme as it assists in clustering a series of related themes.

- Polarization includes exploring for oppositional relationships among emergent themes. Here differences, and not similarities, are examined.

- Contextualization requires the researchers to look for connections among emergent themes by identifying the contextual elements, such as temporal or cultural themes.

- Numeration consists of making a frequency count regarding how often the emergent theme is supported.

- Function involves the researchers examining the emergent themes for their particular function within the transcript.

In this step of searching for connections across emergent themes, the researcher ends with bringing the results of this step together. Smith and colleagues recommend making a graphic representation of the structure of the emergent themes from the transcript.

During IPA analysis, researchers can ask critical questions of the texts from the participants' interviews. Smith and Osborn (2015) suggested the following questions: "What is the person trying to achieve here? Is something leaking out here that wasn't intended? Do I have a sense of something going on here that maybe the participants themselves are less aware of?" (p. 54).

Step 5. Moving to the next case

Now the researchers move on to the next participant's transcript or narrative and repeat the process. Smith et al. (2009) emphasized that researchers need to allow new themes to emerge with each subsequent narrative.

Step 6. Looking for patterns across cases

This is an especially creative task where researchers search for which themes are most potent and how one theme from one narrative aids in illuminating a different narrative. Sometimes this will involve renaming themes or reconfiguring them. At this stage, the analysis reaches a more theoretical level as the researchers now explain that themes or superordinate themes are specific to individual narratives but also represent higher order concepts which narratives share. Smith and colleagues (2009) offered a number of ways the result of this analysis can be presented. A graphic, for instance, can be designed that shows the connections of the themes for the entire group. A table of themes for the entire group of narratives can be constructed illustrating how themes are nested within superordinate themes.

Smith (2011) detailed the concept of a gem as a valuable concept for interpretive phenomenological analysis. He defined a gem as "a singular utterance made by a participant with great resonance across the case and corpus" (Smith, 2017, p. 303). These short passages can have a significance that is completely disproportionate to their size. A gem can provide valuable insight into the experience of a participant. Smith (2011) posited a spectrum of gems from shining, to suggestive, to secret. The first type of a gem he calls shining, where the gem is clearly apparent. Researchers do not need to be especially attentive to see it. In the middle of the spectrum is the suggestive gem that requires some attention by the researchers. The gem is partially present but needs more detective work, as Smith says, to bring it fully forth. A secret gem is the third type and is at the other end of the spectrum. This gem can easily be missed. Researchers need to pay close attention to even notice it. A great deal of detective work is required to bring out the meaning of this utterance.

Smith recently published a study using IPA that provides an example of his methodology (Smith, Spiers, Simpson, & Nicolls, 2017). Twenty-one participants were interviewed to discover their experiences living with an ileostomy. The researchers conducted a detailed, idiographic examination of each case followed by a cross-case comparison of patterns. Themes were clustered together, and two superordinate themes were identified using his techniques of abstraction and subsumption. The first superordinate theme was Ileostomy's intrapersonal impact. Its two subordinate themes were (1) The destabilizing effect of ileostomy on sense of self and (2) Employing illness to positively reframe sense of self. The second superordinate theme was The impact of ileostomy on relationships with others. Its four subordinate themes included Disclosure, Intimate relationships, Relationships with friends, and Family relationships. Smith et al.'s (2017) results were supported with a number of gems.

INTERNATIONAL EXAMPLES OF IPA RESEARCH FROM VARIOUS DISCIPLINES

From the Department of Clinical Speech and Language Studies in Ireland, Moloney and Walshe (2018) investigated the impact of difficulty with swallowing (dysphagia) in persons following stroke using IPA. Data were gleaned from 10 published autobiographical texts written by persons who had experienced a stroke and subsequent dysphagia. IPA resulted in six superordinate themes, each with associated subordinate themes (Table 9.1).

Athletes' experiences of social support during their transition out of elite sport was the focus of a study in the UK (Brown, Webb, Robinson, & Cotgreave, 2018). These researchers designed the study using IPA principles. Eight former elite athletes participated in in-depth interviews. Seven of the eight athletes

TABLE 9.1

Superordinate and Subordinate Themes Associated With Living With Dysphagia Following Stroke

	Superordinate Themes	Subordinate Themes
Living with dysphagia after stroke	Physical consequences of dysphagia	Becoming familiar with the physical consequences of dysphagia Living with the impact of the physical consequences of dysphagia
	Process of recovery	What will the future hold Setting and achieving goals Dealing with setbacks
	Coping and adjusting	Coping strategies Self-management techniques Learning to live with dysphagia
	Changed relationships	Relationship with food and drink Relationship with family Relationship with health care professionals
	Society	Feeling excluded from society Concerns regarding the perceptions of others Reintegrating into society
	Control	Loss of control Helplessness and reliance on others Attempting to regain control (p. 1529)

Source: Reprinted with permission from Moloney, J. & Walshe, M. (2018). "I had no idea what a complicating business eating is . . . ": A qualitative study of the impact of dysphagia during stroke recovery. *Disability and Rehabilitation, 40,* 1524–1531. p. 1529.

had competed at the Olympic Games. Reading of the interview transcripts was informed by five concepts: intersubjectivity, selfhood, temporality, project, and embodiment. Notes were written in three stages when reading the transcripts. In the first stage, attention was directed toward the structure of the participant's experience. The concern of the second stage was the participant's use of language such as repetition of phrases or words, metaphors used, and the manner of how the account was expressed. The third stage consisted of a more interpretive, conceptual level of examining the text to obtain a deeper understanding of the meaning. Aided with these notes, emergent themes were identified and clustered together to identify superordinate themes. This data analysis process was completed separately for each participant. Then a cross-case analysis was done to identify similarities, differences, and patterns linking participants' experiences to achieve higher order concepts. Findings revealed two broad stages of transition for the athletes. In the first stage, two superordinate themes emerged: (1) Feeling cared for and understood and (2) Ability to ask for and seek support. In the second stage of transitioning, a shift in the athletes' self-concept occurred. The superordinate theme was entitled The role of support in transitioning self. Brown et al. (2018) constructed a table to illustrate the process they used in identifying themes from subordinate to superordinate themes.

Using IPA, Allan, Ungar, and Eatough (2018) explored the experiences of couple and family therapists learning an evidence-based approach in working with families and couples. This study took place in Canada and came from the discipline of Education. Three superordinate themes emerged: Supports and challenges in learning, Embodiment of a therapy practice, and Experiences of shame while learning. Allan et al. presented an excellent example of ideography as an important component of interpretive phenomenological analysis. Smith (2011) noted "the pivotal role played by single utterances and small passages of the analysis of a research corpus" (p. 6). He referred to this type of passage as a "gem." Allan and colleagues included this "gem" from their analysis of the theme of shame while learning an evidence-based approach:

> And I'm just like oh my God, that's it, that's it, and then I begin to tell them the story about how I had to put this together through my supervision, the shame piece, my sister's suicide and me feeling responsible and this is what I was hiding inside myself and having that line up with the emotion was incredibly powerful and it was very dysregulating. I was actually pretty dissociated there. (Allan et al., 2018, p. 170)

In Australia from Music Therapy comes an IPA examining how four individuals with mild to moderate dementia experienced a community-based group therapeutic songwriting program (Baker & Stretton-Smith, 2018).

FIGURE 9.1

Steps 1–3 of Interpretative Phenomenological Analysis (IPA). Emergent Themes, Interview Transcript, and Exploratory Comments (from left to right)

Emergent Themes	Interview Transcript	Exploratory Comments
Songwriting was rewarding as it encouraged Nora to reengage in thought and re-enter a 'music world' Songwriting was rewarding as it showed the group's ability to create despite 'disabilities' and diverse levels of musical experience	Interviewer: I'm sure it was a new experience for a lot of people Nora*: Oh, I think so, you know. It's really very um, it's very rewarding because it makes you think again and you come into a music world again. And you play these tunes and then to create something. That was really rewarding for me that we managed, well it's such a different, you know, group of people. But we still managed to create something in a simple way.	**Author** Songwriting is rewarding because it 'makes you think again and come into a music world again' *Use of 'again' (indicating something experienced before)* <u>Rewarding experience of group TSW as a cognitive and creative activity (re-engaging in a thought process and musical process)</u> **Author** Echoes previous comments re: 'managing' to create songs with a 'different group of people'. Describes creating songs with diverse group as an accomplishment and 'rewarding', rather than as a limitation (as alluded to earlier) *Meaning of 'different' – Nora refers to group as 'variety of people with different disabilities' following this statement.* *Repetition of word 'manage' (accomplishment/ability despite disability/lack of songwriting experience).* *Use of 'we' (collective)* <u>TSW as rewarding – surprised at ability and accomplishment of group during TSW process</u>

*descriptive comments = plain font

Linguistic comments = italics

Conceptual comments = underlined

Source: Reprinted with permission from Baker, F. A., & Stretton-Smith. P. A. (2018). Group therapeutic songwriting and dementia: Exploring the perspectives of participants through interpretive phenomenological analysis. *Music Therapy Perspectives, 36,* 50–66. p. 53.

In addition to interviews with these four persons with dementia, three support staff were interviewed. Case by case these interviews were analyzed and then searched for recurrent themes. Baker and Stretton-Smith provided a figure that illustrated the movement from descriptive to linguistic to conceptual exploratory comments about the interview quotes (Figure 9.1). Four recurrent group themes evolved: (1) Therapeutic songwriting enhanced positive self-experiences, (2) Group therapeutic songwriting fostered connection and collaboration, (3) Therapeutic songwriting stimulated learning, cognition, and active language use, and (4) Group context impacted the depth of exploration and sometimes highlighted challenges. The researchers provided sample quotes for all the superordinate themes and are in the supplementary material in the appendix.

Representing Family Medicine in the United States, Nutting and Grafsky (2018) investigated how a person's diagnosis of Crohn's disease affected the couple's relationship and young adult life cycle transitions. IPA was used to analyze individual and couple interviews with five young adult couples in which one of the partners had Crohn's disease. Nutting and Grafsky followed Smith et al.'s (2009) process of exploratory initial coding to identify meanings and language used with three types of coding: descriptive, linguistic, and conceptual. After initial coding was completed, they developed and connected emergent themes. A theme was considered emergent if it had been mentioned in three or more quotes from different participants. Once themes were identified, the researchers then employed abstraction, subsumption, and polarization to finalize the four themes and describe the essence of the couples' experiences: Couples' experiences of diagnosis, Biopsychosocial effects, Relationship functioning and satisfaction, and Interference in life-cycle transitions.

In summary, Smith, Flowers, and Larkin's interpretive phenomenological methodology took center stage in this chapter. To illustrate their approach, international studies conducted by researchers from various disciplines were described. Student study activities can be found in Appendices A and B. In Chapter 10, which follows, Karin Dahlberg's hermeneutic reflective lifeworld research is presented as the final approach of interpretive phenomenology to be covered in this book.

REFERENCES

Allan, R., Ungar, M., & Eatough, V. (2018). "Now I know the terrain": Phenomenological exploration of CFTs learning an evidence-based practice. *Contemporary Family Therapy, 40*, 164–175.

Baker, F. A., & Stretton-Smith, P. A. (2018). Group therapeutic songwriting and dementia: Exploring the perspectives of participants through interpretative phenomenological analysis. *Music Therapy Perspectives, 36*, 50–66.

Brown, C. J., Webb, T. T., Robinson, M. A., & Cotgreave, R. (2018). Athletes' experiences of social support during their transition out of elite sport: An interpretive phenomenological analysis. *Psychology of Sport & Exercise, 36*, 71–80.

Moloney, J., & Walshe, M. (2018). "I had no idea what a complicating business eating is.": A qualitative study of the impact of dysphagia during stroke recovery. *Disability and Rehabilitation, 40*, 1524–1531.

Nutting, R., & Grafsky, E. L. (2018). Crohn's disease and the young couple: An interpretive phenomenological analysis. *Contemporary Family Therapy, 40*, 176–187.

Smith, J. A. (1996). Beyond the divide between cognition and discourse: Using interpretive phenomenological analysis in health psychology. *Psychology and Health, 11*, 261–271.

Smith, J. A. (2011). "We could be diving for pearls": The value of the gem in experiential qualitative psychology. *Qualitative Methods in Psychology Bulletin, 12*, 6–15.

Smith, J. A. (2017). Interpretive phenomenological analysis: Getting at lived experience. *The Journal of Positive Psychology, 12*, 303–304.

Smith, J. A., Flowers, P., & Larkin, M. (2009). *Interpretive phenomenological analysis.* Los Angeles, CA: SAGE.

Smith, J. A. & Osborn, M. (2015). Interpretive phenomenological analysis. In J. A. Smith (Ed.), *Qualitative psychology: A practical guide to methods* (pp. 53–80). London: SAGE.

Smith, J. A., Spiers, J., Simpson, P., & Nicolls, A. R. (2017). The psychological challenges of living with an ileostomy: An interpretative phenomenological analysis. *Health Psychology, 36*, 143–151.

Karin Dahlberg's Hermeneutic Reflective Lifeworld Research Methodology

Chapter 10 revisits Dahlberg, Dahlberg, and Nyström's (2008) reflective lifeworld research, but this time their hermeneutic interpretive approach takes center stage. Two studies conducted by Dahlberg and her colleagues, one on inadequate care in the emergency care units and the second one on aphasia as existential loneliness, are presented. Additional studies by nurse researchers in Sweden are included to help illustrate their hermeneutic methodology. The chapter ends with a comparison of the four interpretive phenomenological approaches addressed in Part III.

....

HERMENEUTIC REFLECTIVE LIFEWORLD METHODOLOGY

Data Analysis

Interpretive methodological principles are based in lifeworld hermeneutics (Dahlberg et al., 2008). Hermeneutic interpretation involves engaging in a dialogue with the text. Dahlberg and colleagues stressed that in neither descriptive analysis, which was the focus of Chapter 6, nor hermeneutic analysis, do researchers follow locked rigid steps. Openness to the phenomenon under study is essential. Ways to proceed for data gathering are essentially the same in their phenomenological and hermeneutic lifeworld research. Differences definitely appear, though, during data analysis. Dahlberg et al.'s descriptive phenomenological analysis aims at describing an essential structure of the phenomenon under study while their hermeneutic analysis involves interpretation, although both are meaning oriented.

Both descriptive phenomenology and hermeneutical traditions are concerned with researchers studying phenomena as they reveal themselves and not with imposing preconceived ideas on them. This openness, however, is based on a scientific and rigorous approach, which differs from an unreflective approach of the natural attitude. In scientific methodological interpretations, the following questions need to be addressed.

- What data are used in the interpretation, and how were they gathered?

- What questions have been asked?

- How has openness been practiced?

- Is a particular comment really an expression of an understanding of the focused phenomenon or is another object in focus?

- How has the relevance of the interpretations been verified?

- (and, perhaps most important) What influence has the researcher's pre-understanding had on the interpretation? (Dahlberg et al., 2008, p. 278)

The researcher begins hermeneutical analysis by reading the texts as a whole to obtain a preliminary understanding of the phenomenon. Dahlberg and colleagues acknowledged that this initial reading does not involve interpretation yet. After this first reading, however, the researchers begin a dialogue with the text to uncover clues about the meaning involved in the text. The researcher actively questions and interrogates the data. For example, the researcher thinks, this passage of the text seems to imply this meaning. Is a similar meaning anywhere else in this text? I am interpreting this passage this way. Is there anything in this text that opposes this interpretation? In dialoguing with the text, Dahlberg et al. (2008) explained that researchers move from viewing the text as an object to something they can converse with. Researchers begin to question the text about what and how it is said, about its content, and about its meaning. Dahlberg and colleagues (2008) provided some examples:

- Is a particular comment really an expression of an understanding of the focused phenomenon or is another object in focus?

- How do the different utterances fit with each other within the framework of a single person's narrative?

- Does the interviewee express more than one understanding?

- If so, do they agree with one another?

- Are there also opposing statements or observations? (p. 253)

Once the researcher has a preliminary understanding of the data, a preliminary structure that includes themes and subthemes can be created to aid in clarification of what meanings are there. Next, searching for hidden meaning can begin. A new interpretive dialogue with the texts occurs, and tentative interpretations are made. The researchers keep going with this dialogue until all the data relevant to the phenomenon under study are covered in the entire data set.

Dahlberg and colleagues (2008) cautioned that interpretation is tentative regarding its validity and must be evaluated prior to going to the next level of abstraction in the hermeneutic spiral. Lifeworld research is governed by the general principles of moving between the whole—the parts—the whole which is central to understanding. As researchers analyze a text for meaning, they must address how each part is understood in regard to the whole and also how the whole is understood in regard to the parts. Tentative interpretations at lower levels of the hermeneutic spiral are the focus of the next phase in Dahlberg et al.'s (2008) interpretive analysis. Here tentative interpretations of each text are compared with one another to develop a comprehensive understanding of the phenomenon under study and a main interpretation. The challenge is to enter at this level of interpretation "upon the thin ice of understanding latent meanings in data in order to develop skills that increase the ability to see, understand and explain structures and patterns that are not fully overt" (p. 282).

Our interpretations provide a background of our pre-understanding. Researchers use this pre-understanding to understand the phenomenon in a new way. Here openness is essential as researchers are critical of these pre-understandings and need to be cautious in treating them in the process of understanding. Prior research or theories can be used in interpretational understandings. Dahlberg et al. (2008) caution that theories should not be used in a predictive manner, and their use in analysis too early can be detrimental to interpretation. Theory has just one purpose, and that is to help researchers see their data and its meaning better.

At Dahlberg et al.'s (2008) higher levels of the hermeneutic spiral, researchers develop a whole new comprehensive understanding of the phenomenon under study and its main interpretation. At this level, a comparative analysis of tentative interpretations is done to identify similarities and differences. Dahlberg et al. use the metaphor of assembling a jigsaw puzzle as the researchers formulate new interpretations that connect prior interpretation to each other. When at this higher level of interpretation, theoretical tools are more predictive than in the lower level of interpretation. A "reasonable" interpretation is one that is comprehensive and also congruent with theories or well-established facts (Dahlberg et al., 2008). Researchers must stay open, however, to the possibility that their understanding may be opposite of previous findings. The main interpretation can be viewed as an umbrella of earlier interpretations. Because in hermeneutical analysis, understanding goes beyond the context given in a specific study, generalizations are possible. In examining the validity of interpretations at higher levels of the hermeneutic spiral, it may be necessary for the researcher to contact the participants in the study to obtain additional data to help with the exploration of the phenomenon.

Dahlberg et al. (2008) offered some criteria for evaluating the validity of tentative interpretations:

- The source of a valid tentative interpretation should be only an actual piece of data. An interpretation that leaves a considerable amount of the same data unexplained is viewed as weak.

- For a valid tentative interpretation there should be no other interpretations that to the same degree or more meaningfully explain the same data.

- There must be no contradictions in the data behind a tentative interpretation that is considered valid. (p. 288)

Hermeneutic Examples of Studies Conducted by Dahlberg and Her Colleagues

Dahlberg et al. (2008) provided hermeneutic examples of their reflective lifeworld research approach. One example was their study of inadequate care in emergency care units (ECU) in Sweden. The research question was, "What are the conditions that explain the provision of inadequate care in an ECU unit with reported problems concerning caring attitudes?" (pp. 289–290). Nine professional caregivers participated in the study. Findings first included eight interpretations that described various aspects of the conditions that were related to the performance of care in the ECU:

- The concept of care has a practical meaning only.

- Caring is organized according to a high degree of division of labor.

- Caring takes place according to fixed schedules and cues.

- A caring attitude needs confirmation from patients.

- Coalitions prevent discussions about how to improve care.

- Medical goals are distinct—caring goals are obscure.

- A critical atmosphere generates feelings of stress in caring situations.

- Medical treatment is highly valued—care is undervalued.

The main interpretation was entitled "The lack of a holistic perspective." The common denominator for all of these eight interpretations was that a holistic approach was lacking. Dahlberg and colleagues described this main interpretation. Some theories were included in connection with the presentation of the interpretations.

Aphasia as existential loneliness was a second study conducted by Dahlberg et al. (2008), included here to provide another illustration of their hermeneutic reflective lifeworld research approach. The purpose was to explore the experiences of aphasia and patients' struggle to regain the ability to communicate. Nine individuals participated in interviews, and three of these persons were involved in follow-up interviews to help with tentative interpretations. Analysis involved comparing and combining themes and subthemes. Next the researchers compared the themes with their written reflections of their pre-understandings. The subthemes were then viewed as pieces to a jigsaw puzzle and no longer were attached to their respective themes. Six interpretations were discovered, and together they explained the meanings identified in their subthemes listed below.

- It is essential to repress feelings in order to act rationally during the acute phase.

- Emotional life is intertwined with the struggle to regain language.

- It is not necessary to name the world in order to recognize its meaning.

- Worrying about being considered stupid.

- Feelings of loneliness creates distance from other people.

- Strategies to handle communication problems help to create distance to the situation.

The main interpretation was "Becoming a symbolic stranger in a previously well-known world is an alienating process" (p. 315). Dahlberg et al. (2008) described this as

The existential meaning of reversible aphasia is that communion, interaction and interpersonal relations become more important than ever before. Strong elements of continuing aphasia is characterized by a life and death struggle to use and/or understand words. Individuals thus affected still, several years after their brain lesion, find themselves excluded from communication when failing to express their thoughts and/or guess the meaning of a conversation. In their struggle for existence they need much more time than they are given to talk and/or to puzzle their fragmented impressions together. During such circumstances it is impossible to direct interest beyond oneself in order to be involved in something other than a struggle for talking and understanding. The existential meaning of continuing severe aphasia is thus characterized by alienation and loneliness, leaving the individual to find a balance between a fight filled with agony and giving up in order to avoid further humiliation. (p. 315–316)

Additional Examples of Dahlberg et al.'s Hermeneutic Reflective Lifeworld Methodology

Nurse researchers in Sweden used Dahlberg et al.'s (2008) hermeneutic reflective lifeworld approach to explore young children's experiences of support during needle-related medical procedures (Karlsson, Englund, Enskär, Nyström, & Rydström, 2016). Participant observation and interviews were held with 21 children between 3 and 7 years of age. After dwelling with the transcribed interviews and viewing the recorded observations, six themes emerged. Interpretations of the themes followed, and as a final interpretive step, the researchers formulated a comprehensive understanding of children's experience of support during needle-related medical procedures. For each theme, different preliminary interpretations were discussed. The interpretation most consistent with the data and the purpose of the study were again tested to make sure there was nothing in the data to contradict this interpretation. To obtain a more comprehensive understanding of the phenomenon being studied, Karlsson et al. repeatedly went back and forth between the whole of the entire dataset, the parts, and the new whole of understanding to make certain of the internal consistency of the final interpretation. The following six themes were discovered: Being the center of attention, Getting help with distraction, Being pampered, Being involved, Entrusting oneself to the safety of adults, and Being rewarded.

A second example of the interpretive reflective lifeworld approach was provided by Svanström, Andersson, Rosén, and Berglund (2016). In Sweden, the purpose of this study was to examine experiences of staff implementing a learning supportive model to increase patient involvement and autonomy in care in a hemodialysis center. Staff wrote stories when participations felt successful in supporting patients when learning to use the model and also situations when they felt unsuccessful. Open-ended interviews, notes from group supervision sessions, and monthly reflective meetings were other sources of data collected. Using the hermeneutic reflective lifeworld approach, the researchers were in a continuous dialogue with the data as meaning units from the data were unpacked. Next, clusters of meanings were built and used as a background to develop a new text divided into themes. As the final step, Svanström et al. wrote a comprehensive interpretation that included the themes, clusters of meanings, and data as background while concentrating on the changes in experiences and attitudes of the staff during the implementation of this model of care. This interpretation became the third theme called Changes achieved through the project. The other two themes were Intent to change approach and Importance of supervision and reflection. An excerpt from the interpretation of the changes theme is presented here:

> From an initial feeling that changing was a difficult task, the participants moved to understanding the model and embracing it during dialogue with patients and when reflecting on their experiences during supervision sessions. The experience of implementing the model has, from the staff's perspective, not been easy but has led to increased self-confidence and feelings of deepened competence in dialogue with patients. Staff also perceived increased patient involvement and patient autonomy in hemodialysis care in the unit. (Svanström et al., 2016, p. 7)

Dahlberg et al. (2008) called for qualitative studies to be more rigorous. They warned that studies with weak philosophical and epistemological underpinnings can end up in a "mishmash of methods." They went on to assert that

> Phenomenology, hermeneutics and the reflective lifeworld research approach offer a consistent epistemology that form a solid basis for research, a firm foundation that prevents the researcher from scientific malpractice at the same time as it preserves the richness and beauty of the lifeworld. (p. 350)

In Table 10.1 can be found a listing of the steps involved in the four interpretive phenomenological methods covered in Part III.

TABLE 10.1

Comparison of Four Interpretive Phenomenological Methods

van Manen	Benner	Smith, Flowers, & Larkin	Dahlberg, Dahlberg, & Nyström
Hermeneutic phenomenological reflection	Developing lines of inquiry and examining modes of engagement	Reading & rereading the first case. Initial noting - Descriptive comments - Linguistic comments - Conceptual comments	Initial reading of the texts as a whole to obtain preliminary understanding of the phenomenon (no interpretation yet)
Conducting thematic analysis - Wholistic or sententious approach - Selective or highlighted approach - Detailed or line-by-line approach	Undergo critical reflective exercises of researcher's biases & assumptions to create openness	Developing emergent themes	Begin dialogue with the text to uncover clues about meaning involved in text
Gleaning thematic descriptions from artistic sources	Choose sources of text & sample of situations such as individual or group interviews, participant observation, videotapes, documents, & media	Searching for connections across emergent themes	Create a preliminary structure which includes themes & subthemes to aid in clarification of meanings

Interpretation through conversation
 	
Collaborative analysis: the research seminar/group
	Interpretive dialogue begins with first interview, so data collection & analysis are not separated
	
	Multiple interviews are preferred for interpretation with participants
		Moving to the next case
		
		Looking for patterns across cases:
		  - Superordinate themes
		  - Subordinate themes
			Search for hidden meaning and new interpretive dialogue with texts as one moves between the whole and the parts. Tentative interpretations made at lower levels of hermeneutic spiral

Determining incidental and essential themes
 	
Hermeneutic phenomenological writing
 	
Attending to the speaking of language
 	
Varying the examples
 	
Maintaining pedagogical relation to the phenomena
	Uncover commonalities & differences in meanings & understanding. Five sources of commonality:
	  - Situation
	  - Embodiment
	  - Temporality
	  - Concerns
	  - Common meanings
			Prior research or theories can be used in interpretational understandings but not in a predictive way

(*Continued*)

TABLE 10.1 (Continued)

van Manen	Benner	Smith, Flowers, & Larkin	Dahlberg, Dahlberg, & Nyström
Balancing the research context by considering the parts as a whole	Interpretive processes focus on analysis of specific incidents		At higher levels of hermeneutic spiral, new comprehensive understanding of the phenomenon & its main interpretation are developed
	Use of 3 interrelated interpretive strategies: - Paradigm cases - Exemplars - Thematic analysis moving back & forth between parts of text and whole		Theoretical tools are more predictive at this higher level of interpretation
			Researchers need to stay open to their pre-understanding & be cautious in the process of understanding

COMPARISON OF THE FOUR INTERPRETIVE PHENOMENOLOGICAL METHODOLOGIES

van Manen (1990) and Benner (1994) called for multiple interviews with each participant to facilitate interpretation. van Manen's is the only approach that includes collaborative interpretation with a research seminar or group. Benner and van Manen both focus on lived body (corporeality) and lived time (temporality) in reflecting on the essential meaning of an experience. Dahlberg et al.'s (2008) analysis progresses through levels of the hermeneutic spiral. Benner (1994) uses the three interrelated interpretive strategies of paradigm cases, exemplars, and thematic analysis. van Manen (1990) called for conducting thematic analysis in three options: wholistic, selective, or detailed. He differentiates between essential and incidental themes while Smith, Flowers, and Larkin (2009) categorized themes into superordinate and subordinate themes. Smith et al.'s methodology is the only one that divides up initial notes into descriptive, linguistic, and conceptual comments. Only in van Manen's (1990) approach are developing themes supplemented by artistic sources such as poetry, lyrics, and art.

CHOOSING ONE OF THE INTERPRETIVE PHENOMENOLOGICAL METHODOLOGIES

van Manen's methodology appeals to researchers who are attracted to being able to use various artistic sources such as song lyrics or artwork to help with thematic description. Benner also invites researchers to think outside the box in data collection. She suggests allowing participants to take their own photographs of their experiences to supplement their interviews. Benner's approach includes the use of multiple interviews with each participant. The researcher then needs to be able to return repeatedly to the sample participants for interpretation. The larger the total amount of text, the more opportunity it permits for redundancy and clarification. It also is a bias control strategy. Benner encourages small-group interviews if this is a possibility for a researcher. In Benner's approach, she does call for expert and consensual validation of a subset of the data to ensure meanings are supported by the text. A researcher then would need to have an expert or two to validate a subset of the data. If researchers know they will not be able to conduct multiple interviews with participants, then Benner's approach may not be the best fit.

Smith (2010) compared his approach with Giorgi's methodology. Smith explained that in contrast to Giorgi's general structure of the phenomenon being studied, his IPA (interpretative phenomenological analysis) focuses on microanalysis of each individual's experience. What focus does a researcher want in choosing a methodology? This would help to decide which phenomenological approach to use.

Compared to Dahlberg et al.'s approach, Smith and colleagues' analysis is more structured. Smith et al. (2009) call for dividing transcripts into descriptive, linguistic, and conceptual comments. Dahlberg et al.'s approach is more open and flexible. In making your choice, you need to remember that one methodology is not better than the other. It depends on what fits best with your particular research question and sample.

In summary, Dahlberg and colleagues' hermeneutic reflective lifeworld approach was the focus of this chapter, which concludes Part III of this book. Examples of studies conducted in Sweden were described to illustrate their approach. Possible reasons for choosing one of the interpretive phenomenological methodologies over another were discussed. Remember that in Appendices A and B you can find student study activities. Part IV, Evaluating, Writing, and Teaching Phenomenology, begins with Chapter 11, which focuses attention on the trustworthiness of phenomenological research.

REFERENCES

Benner, P. (Ed.) (1994). *Interpretive phenomenology: Embodiment, caring and ethics in health and illness.* Thousand Oaks, CA: SAGE.

Dahlberg, K., Dahlberg, H., & Nyström, M. (2008). *Reflective lifeworld research.* Lund, Sweden: Studentlitteratur.

Karlsson, K., Englund, A. C. D., Enskär, K., Nyström, M., & Rydström, I. (2016). Experiencing support during needle-related medical procedures: A hermeneutic study with young children (3–7 years). *Journal of Pediatric Nursing, 31,* 667–677.

Smith, J. A. (2010). Interpretive phenomenological analysis: A reply to Amedeo Giorgi. *Existential Analysis, 21,* 186–192.

Smith, J. A., Flowers, P., & Larkin, M. (2009). *Interpretive phenomenological analysis.* Los Angeles, CA: SAGE.

Svanström, R., Andersson, S., Rosén, H., & Berglund, M. (2016). Moving from theory to practice: Experience of implementing a learning supporting model designed to increase patient involvement and autonomy in care. *BMC Research Notes, 9:*361. doi.10.1186? s13104-016-2165-5

van Manen, M. (1990). *Researching lived experience.* London, Ontario, Canada: The State University of New York.

PART IV

Evaluating, Writing, and Teaching Phenomenology

Trustworthiness in Qualitative Research

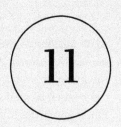

In this chapter, the rigor involved in qualitative studies is the focus. It doesn't matter whether a study is a descriptive or an interpretive phenomenological study. It doesn't matter whose methodology was chosen to guide the study. A rigorous research design is essential if qualitative researchers do not want their research to reflect method slurring. Qualitative researchers must, however, walk a fine line between the quest for rigor and not sacrificing creativity or insightfulness, which are hallmarks of qualitative research. If qualitative scholars use a one-size-fits-all formula for analyzing their data, as Morse (2006) warned, qualitative findings can be "perfectly healthy but dead" (p. 98). Rigor involves fidelity to the spirit of qualitative work, and if the spirit of qualitative inquiry is squelched, instead of rigor we might get rigor mortis (Sandelowski, 1993). The ongoing debate on which terms should be used, trustworthiness versus reliability and validity, is discussed in this chapter. Criteria and strategies for enhancing the trustworthiness of qualitative research are addressed. Two guides specific to evaluating the rigor of a phenomenological study are detailed. In addition, other criteria for enhancing evaluate qualitative research in general are included. The chapter concludes with an exercise that faculty can assign their students regarding evaluating a phenomenological study.

....

TRUSTWORTHINESS VS. RELIABILITY AND VALIDITY

Debate currently is ongoing regarding the terms that should be used in assessing the rigor in qualitative research. The terms reliability and validity are shunned by some researchers who hold them as being associated with quantitative research and the postpositivist paradigm. Because the assumptions and goals of qualitative research are different from those in quantitative research, some qualitative researchers advocate the use of different terms to evaluate qualitative research. Other qualitative researchers, however, defend the use of the quantitative terms of reliability and validity, which are mainstream and can be used by all researchers. These terms are also recognizable for quality by funding agencies in their decision making.

Criteria to evaluate standards in qualitative research are particularly challenging due to the need to methodologically conduct a rigorous study but not, however, to the exclusion of creativity. Lincoln and Guba (1985) developed a parallel perspective for evaluating qualitative research. Their overall standard of trustworthiness consists of four criteria parallel to the quantitative criteria of internal validity, reliability, objectivity, and external validity. Credibility relates to the confidence one can have in the truth of the findings. Credibility is parallel to internal validity. The second criterion of Lincoln and Guba is dependability, which refers to the stability of the findings over time and conditions. You cannot have credibility without dependability. It is equated with reliability. Confirmability parallels objectivity and focuses on agreement between two or more persons regarding the meaning and accuracy of the data. Keeping an audit trail of your decisions during data analysis is helpful. Akin to generalizability in quantitative research is transferability, which addresses the applicability of findings to other contexts. Here the researcher provides enough thick description to enable a person considering making a transfer to be able to decide if it is possible. Guba and Lincoln (1994) added one additional criterion of authenticity to the framework. It refers to the degree to which a researcher faithfully reports the range of realities of the experiences of the participants.

Morse (2015a) called for returning to the terminology of social science that was used four decades ago prior to Lincoln and Guba's (1985) criteria. Morse recommends going back to using the term "rigor" in place of trustworthiness and replacing dependability, credibility, and transferability with reliability, validity, and generalizability, respectively. Morse developed a table summarizing her recommendations for strategies for achieving validity and reliability in qualitative research (Table 11.1). Morse makes the case that member checking is of little value in determining validity or achieving reliability. Regarding coding systems and inter-rater reliability, Morse argued these are appropriate only in semistructured interviews and not in unstructured interviews.

While Morse (2015a) is against member checking, Munhall (1994) is on the other side of this qualitative debate. Munhall stressed that in a phenomenological study it is critical for researchers to return to their participants since they are the only persons who will know if you captured the meaning of the experience for them. Munhall explained that the description of the findings may not fully represent the meaning for each participant. Participants should see themselves somewhere in your description of the findings but not

TABLE 11.1

Summary of Recommendations for Strategies for Establishing Rigor in Qualitative Inquiry

Strategy	Validity	Reliability
Prolonged engagement	Yes: for research using observation	No
Thick description	Yes: for research using unstructured interviews	More opportunity for replication of data
Triangulation	Yes: for mixed-method research	No
Development of a coding system and inter-rater reliability	Yes: only for semistructured interview research	Yes: essential for semistructured interview research and multiple coders
Researcher bias	May be evident in research question and design (groups not equivalent, etc.) Data will correct themselves if researcher is responsive to the principles of induction	Not a reliability concern
Negative case analysis	Yes: for research using unstructured interviews With semistructured interviews, attend to missing responses	Not used as a reliability measure
Peer review/ debriefing	Yes: may assist with conceptualization	Not used
Member checking	Not used	Not used
External audits	Not routinely used	Not routinely used

Source: Reprinted with permission from Morse, J. M. (2015). Critical analysis of strategies for determining rigor in qualitative inquiry. *Qualitative Health Research*, 25, 1212–1222, p. 1220.

necessarily in every piece of the description. This is why Munhall recommended that phenomenologists use the word "however" in their writing. You can write that some participants, however, have experienced a different meaning regarding the experience and that there were variations in the situated contexts.

STRATEGIES FOR ENHANCING QUALITY

Polit and Beck (2017) have organized strategies for enhancing quality in qualitative research according to different phases of a research study (Table 11.2). In the table, the strategies are mapped onto Lincoln and Guba's (1985) criteria for evaluation qualitative research. These strategies can include the following:

- Prolonged engagement involves the researcher investing sufficient time in data collection to permit an in-depth understanding of the phenomenon under study.

- Persistent observation refers to the researcher concentrating on relevant aspects of the phenomenon.

- Triangulation involves using multiple sources of data and/or multiple methods of data collection.

- Member checking refers to the researcher obtaining feedback from participants on a draft of the findings in order to allow them the opportunity to review and comment.

- Negative case analysis involves researchers searching for cases that seem to disconfirm their earlier hypothesis or interpretations in order to refine the results.

- Peer debriefing refers to sessions the researcher has with peers to review the findings. Peers can involve persons with expertise in the clinical area of the phenomenon being studied or experts in the methodology, such as phenomenology.

- Inquiry audits involve having an external reviewer carefully review all of the documents, data, and audit trail.

Data saturation is an important aspect of rigor in qualitative inquiry. Morse (2015b) defined data saturation as "the building of rich data within the process of inquiry, by attending to scope and replication, hence in turn, building the theoretical aspects of inquiry" (p. 587). Morse warned that saturation doesn't mean a researcher saturates the specific details of the individual event but rather the characteristics within themes or categories that evolved from analysis are

TABLE 11.2

Quality-Enhancement Strategies in Relation to Lincoln & Guba's Criteria for Trustworthiness

Strategy	Criteria				
	Dependability	Confirmability	Transferability	Credibility	Authenticity
Throughout the Inquiry					
Reflexivity/reflexive journaling				X	X
Careful documentation, audit trail	X	X			
Data Generation					
Prolonged engagement				X	X
Persistent observation				X	X
Comprehensive field notes			X	X	
Theoretically driven sampling				X	
Audio recording and verbatim transcription				X	X
Triangulation (data, method)	X			X	
Saturation of data			X	X	
Member checking	X			X	

(Continued)

TABLE 11.2 (Continued)

Strategy	Criteria				
Data Coding/Analysis					
Transcription rigor				X	
Intercoder checks; development of a codebook		X		X	
Quasi-statistics				X	
Triangulation (investigator, theory, analysis)		X		X	
Search for confirming evidence		X	X	X	
Search for disconfirming evidence/negative case analysis				X	
Peer review/debriefing		X		X	
Inquiry audit	X	X			
Presentation of Findings					
Documentation of quality-enhancement efforts			X	X	
Thick, vivid description			X	X	X
Impactful, evocative writing					X
Disclosure of researcher credentials, background				X	
Documentation of reflexivity				X	

Source: Adapted with permission Polit, D. F., & Beck, C. T. (2017). *Nursing Research: Generating and Assessing Evidence for Nursing Practice.* Philadelphia; PA: Wolters Kluwers. p. 562.

saturated. The more abstract these characteristics are, the more varied the examples may be. Morse went on to explain that common information from participants builds in the shape of a curve. She stressed that qualitative researchers give data at the tails of the curve equal importance. Data need to be specifically collected at these tails to ensure that the risk does not occur that "the data in the center of the curve will overwhelm the less common data, and we will ignore the equally significant data at the tails" (Morse, 2015b, p. 587).

CRITERIA FOR EVALUATING PHENOMENOLOGICAL RESEARCH

First in this section two guides specific to phenomenology are described followed by others that speak to quality criteria for qualitative research in general. Munhall (1994) developed a guide for specifically evaluating the rigor of a phenomenological study. Her criteria included one P and 10 Rs. The one P represents the phenomenological nod that occurs when persons reading or hearing a study's findings nod in agreement. The criteria of the 10 Rs for rigor include the following:

- Resonancy: The findings resonate with people.

- Reasonableness: The interpretation appears reasonable and is a possible explanation of the meaning of an experience.

- Representativeness: The various dimensions of the experience are adequately represented.

- Recognizability: Persons who have not had the experience can recognize certain aspects of it that they are now aware of.

- Raised consciousness: This is a response to reading the study where individuals gain an understanding of an experience they had not previously considered.

- Readability: When the individual reads a phenomenological study, it should read like an interesting conversation.

- Relevance: The study should be relevant to human science and bring us closer to our humanness.

- Revelations: Here some part of an experience that was concealed is now revealed, and a deeper level of understanding is achieved.

- Responsibility: Here researchers are aware of the ethical considerations in conducting their study.

In assessing the quality of phenomenological research, Smith (2011a) described two types of quality. The first type is mainly focused on evaluation that concerns the rigor and evidence base of the qualitative study. In Table 11.3, Smith (2011b) described the core features of a high-quality interpretative phenomenological paper, which can provide a guide to evaluating published papers. Some of these core features include the paper having a clear focus, strong data, rigorous method, elaboration of each theme, and reporting both convergence and divergence. The second measure of quality focuses on the particulars and if "gems" have been identified in the study.

TABLE 11.3

What Makes a Good Interpretative Phenomenological Analysis (IPA) Paper?

The paper should have a clear focus. Papers providing detail of a particular aspect rather than a broad reconnaissance are more likely to be of high quality.

The paper will have strong data. Most IPA is derived from interviews, and this means that, for the most part, getting good data requires doing good interviewing. This is a particular skill that must not be underestimated. The quality of the interview data obtained sets a cap on how good a paper can subsequently be. High-quality data are integral to the success of the papers.

The paper should be rigorous. One should aim to give some measure of prevalence for a theme, and the corpus should be well represented in the analysis. Extracts should be selected to give some indication of convergence and divergence, representativeness and variability. This way the reader gets to see the breadth and depth of the theme. For papers with small sample sizes (1–3), each theme should be supported with extracts from each participant. For papers with sample sizes of 4 to 8, in general, extracts from half the participants should be provided as evidence. For larger sample sizes, researchers should give illustrations from at least three or four participants per theme and also provide some indication of how prevalence of a theme is determined. The overall corpus should also be proportionately sampled. In other words, the evidence base, when assessed in the round, should not be drawn from just a small portion of participants.

Sufficient space must be given to the elaboration of each theme. In certain circumstances, it may well be better to present a subset of the emergent themes so there is room to do justice to each, rather than presenting all themes but doing so superficially.

The analysis should be interpretative, not just descriptive. An interpretive commentary should follow each of the extracts presented. The author is thereby showing the particular ways extracts are contributing to the unfolding theme. In order to do this, the researcher is engaging in the double hermeneutic: trying to make sense of the participant and trying to make sense of participant experience.

The analysis should be pointing to both convergence and divergence. Where an IPA study reports data from more than one participant, there should be a skillful demonstration of both patterns of similarity among participants as well as the uniqueness of the individual experience. The unfolding narrative for a theme thus provides a careful interpretive analysis of how participants manifest the same theme in particular and different ways. This nuanced capturing of similarity and difference, convergence and divergence, is the hallmark of good IPA work.

The paper needs to be carefully written. Good qualitative work always requires good writing. Readers will feel engaged by a well-wrought, sustained narrative and will consider they have learned in detail about the participants' experience of the phenomenon under investigation.

Source: Adapted with permission from Smith, J. A. (2011b). Evaluating the contribution of interpretive phenomenological analysis. *Health Psychology Review, 5*, 9–27, p. 24.

CRITERIA FOR EVALUATING QUALITATIVE RESEARCH IN GENERAL

There are myriad proposed criteria for evaluating qualitative research in general. One example is highlighted here. Whittemore, Chase, and Mandle (2001) developed a synthesis of validity criteria gleaned from earlier published qualitative criteria. They organized the synthesis into primary criteria, which include credibility, authenticity, integrity, and criticality and secondary criteria of vividness, creativity, explicitness, thoroughness, and congruence. In Table 11.4 are specific questions Whittemore et al. suggest using to assess their primary and secondary validity criteria.

In summary, this chapter presented criteria and strategies for enhancing the trustworthiness of qualitative research. Two guides specific to evaluating the rigor of a phenomenological study were included along with other criteria to evaluate qualitative research in general. An exercise was provided that faculty can use to give their students practice in evaluating a phenomenological study. Chapter 12 attention will focus on writing phenomenological studies.

TABLE 11.4

Whittemore & Colleagues' Assessment of Primary and Secondary Criteria of Validity

Criteria	Assessment
Primary criteria Credibility	Do the results of the research reflect the experience of participants or the context in a believable way?
Authenticity	Does a representation of the emic perspective exhibit awareness to the subtle differences in the voices of all participants?
Criticality	Does the research process demonstrate evidence of critical appraisal?
Integrity	Does the research reflect recursive and repetitive checks of validity as well as a humble presentation of findings?
Secondary criteria Explicitness	Have methodological decisions, interpretations, and investigator biases been addressed?
Vividness	Have thick and faithful descriptions been portrayed with artfulness and clarity?
Creativity	Have imaginative ways of organizing, presenting, and analyzing data been incorporated?
Thoroughness	Do the findings convincingly address the questions posed through completeness and saturation?
Congruence	Are the process and the findings congruent? Do all of the themes fit together? Do findings fit into a context outside the study situation?
Sensitivity	Has the investigation been implemented in ways that are sensitive to the nature of human, cultural, and social contexts?

Source: Reprinted with permission from Whittemore, R., Chase, S. K., & Mandle, C. L. (2001). Validity in qualitative research. *Qualitative Health Research, 11*, 522–537. p. 534.

STUDENT EXERCISE FOR EVALUATING A PHENOMENOLOGICAL STUDY

Choose a phenomenological study published by researchers in your discipline. It can be either a descriptive or an interpretive phenomenological study. Then answer the following questions regarding your chosen study:

1. Did the study include a section on rigor/trustworthiness and efforts made to enhance the quality of the study?

2. Was a specific guide for addressing the rigor of the study used? For example, Guba and Lincoln, Whittemore et al., Munhall?

3. What specific strategies did the researchers use to enhance the quality of their phenomenological study?

4. Did these strategies address credibility, dependability, confirmability, transferability, and authenticity?

5. If you were to conduct this phenomenological study, are there any quality enhancement strategies you would use to increase the trustworthiness that were not used in this published study?

6. Based on the information presented in the article of your chosen study, what do you conclude about the study's rigor/trustworthiness?

REFERENCES

Guba, E. G., & Lincoln, Y. S. (1994). Competing paradigms in qualitative research. In N. Denzin & Y. Lincoln (Eds.), *Handbook of qualitative research* (pp. 105–117). Thousand Oaks, CA: SAGE.

Lincoln, Y. S., & Guba, E. G. (1985). *Naturalistic inquiry.* Newbury Park, CA: SAGE.

Morse, J. M. (2006). Insight, inference, evidence, and verification: Creating a legitimate discipline. *International Journal of Qualitative Methods, 5,* 93–100.

Morse, J. M. (2015a). Critical analysis of strategies for determining rigor in qualitative inquiry. *Qualitative Health Research, 25,* 1212–1222.

Morse, J. M. (2015b). Data were saturated . . . *Qualitative Health Research, 25,* 587–588.

Munhall, P. L. (1994). *Revisioning phenomenology: Nursing and health science research.* New York, NY: NLN Press.

Polit, D. F., & Beck, C. T. (2017). *Nursing research: Generating and assessing evidence for nursing practice.* Philadelphia, PA: Wolters Kluwers.

Sandelowski, M. (1993). Rigor or rigor mortis: The problem of rigor in qualitative research revisited. *Advances in Nursing Science, 16,* 108.

Smith, J. A. (2011a). "We could be diving for pearls": The value of the gem in experiential qualitative psychology. *Qualitative Methods in Psychology Bulletin, 12,* 6–15.

Smith, J. A. (2011b). Evaluating the contribution of interpretative phenomenological analysis. *Health Psychology Review, 5,* 9–27.

Whittemore, R., Chase, S. K., & Mandle, C. L. (2001). Validity in qualitative research. *Qualitative Health Research, 11,* 522–537.

Phenomenological Writing

No matter which method you choose to conduct your descriptive or interpretive phenomenological study, the next step is disseminating your findings. In this chapter, approaches to writing a phenomenological study are the focus. The chapter concludes with examples of figures used in some of my published phenomenological studies.

Analysis for themes is a cornerstone in phenomenology, but as van Manen (2014) points out, the real analysis occurs in writing the phenomenological text itself. Phenomenological research cannot be separated from phenomenological writing. Through phenomenological writing "the reader must be taken, touched, overcome by the phenomenological effect of reflective engagement with lived experience" (van Manen, 2014, p. 390).

Writing and rewriting are like an artistic activity where the sculptor or painter creates an artwork by going back to it again and again and again until it is finished. van Manen (2014) asked, "What does it mean to write phenomenologically?" (p. 357). He answered by saying that phenomenological writing starts with wonder in the author and also induces wonder in the reader. Writing is a solitary activity where the writer leaves the ordinary world that one shares with others. The writer steps into what van Manen calls the textorium, which is the world of the text. A phenomenological text should "infect the reader with a sudden realization of the unsuspected enigmatic nature of ordinary reality. . . . Wonder is that moment of being when one is overcome by awe or perplexity—such as when something familiar has turned profoundly unfamiliar" (van Manen, 2014, p. 360).

The expressive method of the vocative, having a text "speak" to readers, is the most challenging aspect of phenomenological research but also the most neglected aspect (van Manen, 2014). Writing is a poetizing activity. van Manen, though, makes clear that poetizing is not the same as making verses in poetry. It is bringing the original experiences to a more primal sense helping the description of the experience to reverberate in the world.

Lived-thoroughness, nearness, intensification, appeal, and epiphany are features of phenomenological writing (van Manen, 2014). Lived-thoroughness refers to a text that vividly brings an experience to the reader. Concrete images, experiential descriptions, and anecdotal examples can be used to achieve this. Once the experience is brought vividly to the readers, then they can reflect phenomenologically on it, which is nearness. Intensification refers to the writer's use of key words to allow the meaning of the experience to come through. Epiphany is the dimension of phenomenological writing that provides a transforming effect on readers where they suddenly grasp the meaning of the experience and it stirs them at the core of their being. Yet another important characteristic of phenomenological writing is vividness. Gadamer (1986) stressed vividness "sets our intuitive capacities in motion" (p. 162). Ricoeur (1991) declared that the text is the place where words amass depth of meaning, "The world of the text is therefore not the world of everyday language. . . . New possibilities of being-in-the-world are opened up within everyday reality" (p. 86).

In discussing approaches to writing phenomenologically, Eisner (1998) claimed that as qualitative researchers we display our signature and that we should just use first person. He continued to say that using first person makes it clear to a reader that a person and not a machine was behind all written words. Our words as the author of a qualitative study must reveal what words can never say. Voices of our participants must be heard in all text. Eisner suggested that metaphors, alliteration, and cadences are as much a part of our toolkit as statistics are in quantitative research. Qualitative authors need to paint in text so that a powerful visual image is generated. Artistry is required as researchers treat the participants' descriptions of the experiences of a phenomenon. Eisner challenges qualitative researchers to infuse their manuscripts with a feeling of energy that is palpable through their words.

....

STRATEGIES

An anecdotal narrative is a common methodological device in phenomenological writing. "Phenomenology tries to penetrate the layers of meaning of the concrete by tilling and turning the soil of daily existence. Anecdote is one of the implements for laying bare the covered-over meanings" (van Manen, 1990, p. 119), and its value in phenomenological writing lies in its power.

Another strategy for presenting qualitative findings is the use of a metaphor. Richardson (1994), introduced metaphor this way:

A literary device, metaphor is the backbone of social science writing. Like the spine, it bears weight, permits movement, is buried beneath the surface, and links parts together into a functional coherent whole. As this metaphor about metaphor suggests, the essence of metaphor is the experiencing and understanding of one thing in terms of another. This is accomplished through comparison. (p. 519)

If a decision is made to use a metaphor, its details need to be carried throughout the analysis and interpretation. The metaphor should be woven throughout the findings. A researcher needs to be aware that depending on the metaphor chosen, there is the possibility that the results are oversimplified and a complex experience is portrayed as trite.

In writing up a phenomenological study, there is a craft in regard to quotes. Sandelowski (1994) identified common errors that researchers make in their articles when it comes to including the participants' quotes. These errors involved using too many quotes to illustrate one idea or theme or just listing one quote after another without any appropriate introduction to the quote. It is important how quotes are introduced into the text of a manuscript. The reader needs to know the context surrounding a specific quote. Why did the researcher choose that particular quote to help bring alive a theme? Quotes can be used for various purposes such as to illustrate ideas, support researcher's claims, to arouse emotion, and to enhance experience (Sandelowski, 1994). One practice that should be avoided is just listing one quote after another without any introduction to each quote.

Morse (2010) implored qualitative writers to avoid "cherry picking." She explained that this happens when writing from thin data. Here only the best quotes are included in an article. Because the researcher has minimal data, the lack of available quotes quickly is depleted from the dataset. Morse made a plea for qualitative researchers to increase sample size to ensure certainty of their findings. Sandelowski (1998) offered some strategies for re-presenting qualitative data. Templates such as time, prevalence, and sensitizing concepts and coding families can be used to successfully disseminate qualitative findings in a research report.

Graff and Birkenstein (2018) shared some sage advice on the art of quoting. They invite us to see quotations as "orphan words that have been taken from their original contexts and that need to be integrated into their new textual surroundings" (p. 44). They continue that in framing a quotation the writer should think of it as a "quotation sandwich with the statement introducing it serving as the top slice of bread and the explanation following it serving as the bottom slice" (p. 47). Graff and Birkenstein encourage writers to avoid what they term "hit and run quotations", where they insert a quote into a text without framing it.

Thorne and Darbyshire (2005) poked some fun at some problematic patterns in writing and reporting qualitative findings (Table 12.1).

TABLE 12.1

Problematic Patterns in Writing and Reporting Qualitative Findings

Apples and Tuesdays	This is a form of thematic confusion in which the researcher fails in the write-up to interpret and represent parts of the findings in relation to each other. It often results from a failure to recall what precisely was the original research question combined with an enthusiasm for new issues that arose in the course of the inquiry.
Delusions of intimacy	This is a form of what our anthropological ancestors might have termed "going native," in that it suggests an overidentification of the researcher with the researched. Excessive reference to how much "my participants have entrusted me . . . ," "my special relationship" with them, and other forms of special pleading might be suggestive of fuzzy boundaries between the researcher and his or her findings.
The Holy Grail	In this pattern, the researcher assumes that new observations represent important and transferable truths. It usually reflects an overestimation of the meaning that can credibly be extracted from qualitative studies, particularly smaller ones.
In actual fact	This pattern reflects accidental slippage off the constructivist platform on which qualitative inquiries are built. In the worst instances, those afflicted fall directly in a quagmire of realist claims.
Obfuscation	In this pattern, the researcher writes in a manner that is dense and obscure, mistaking situating and languaging for complex thinking.
Bloodless findings	In this pattern, the researcher plays it safe in writing up the research findings, reporting the obvious possibly the most thinly "salami-sliced" "findings" articles, failing to apply any inductive analytic spin to the sequence, structure, or form of the findings.

Source: Reprinted with permission from Thorne, S., & Darbyshire, P. (2005). Land mines in the field: A model proposal for improving the craft of qualitative health research. *Qualitative Health Research, 15,* 1105–1113. p. 1109.

They called these problems land mines in the field that qualitative writers need to avoid stepping on, such as bloodless findings and the Holy Grail. Their catchy titles do help get the attention of researchers to these difficulties in writing qualitative results that researchers need to stay clear of.

Maintaining confidentiality of participants in a qualitative article is of utmost importance since phenomenological studies typically have small sample sizes. Sometimes omitting or changing details of participants may be necessary to help disguise who they are. For instance, instead of saying the participant was 27 years old and lived in Tolland, CT, you could say the participant was in her 20s and lived in New England.

FIGURES

Part of the special relationship to language is the art of using figures or diagrams not only to help summarize key findings of a phenomenological study but also to bring the results to life. For readers of a phenomenological study, a figure or diagram helps to break up page after page of text. Another advantage of using figures and diagrams is to help with meeting the page limitations of a journal where you are submitting your manuscript. Most journals do not count references, tables, or figures in their maximum number of pages. Another benefit of figures or diagrams is that they help to open up more space in your manuscript to provide important details of your methodology. Novice qualitative researchers oftentimes use more space to describe their results to the detriment of describing their methodology. If your methodology appears weak because you haven't included important details in your manuscript, journal reviewers may decide not to recommend your manuscript for publication.

A few examples of incorporating figures in a manuscript are provided here from my published phenomenological studies. Figure 12.1 is a figure I used in my study entitled "The Impact of Birth Trauma on Breastfeeding: A Tale of Two Pathways" (Beck & Watson, 2008). Eight themes emerged from mothers' descriptions. Three of the eight themes propelled mothers to persevere in breastfeeding while five themes led to distressing impediments that hindered women's attempts to breastfeed. I chose to display these eight themes as weights on a breastfeeding scale. Depending on the number and strength of the weights, a mother's experience could tip the breastfeeding scale in one direction or the other.

Figure 12.2 is from my study entitled "Posttraumatic Stress Disorder Due to Childbirth: The Aftermath" (Beck, 2004a). Here I added images and photos beside each of the five themes. As illustrated by the theme titles in this figure, writers of a phenomenological study should strive to have theme titles that have "grab." Creative titles of both themes and the actual title of the study help capture the interest of persons in reading your article. An example of a title

FIGURE 12.1
Breastfeeding Scale

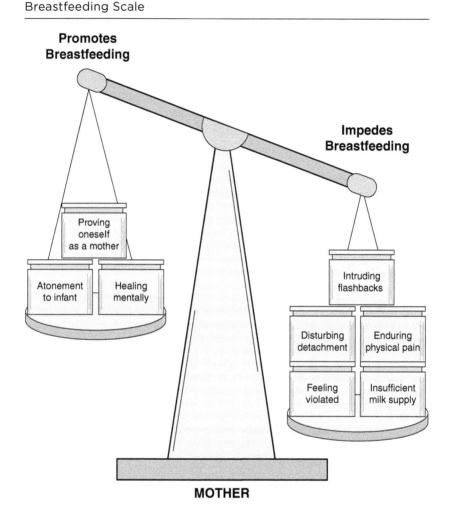

Source: Reprinted with permission from Beck, C. T., & Watson,S (2008). The impact of birth trauma on breastfeeding: A tale of two pathways. *Nursing Research, 57*, 228–236. p. 232.

of one of my phenomenological studies was "Birth Trauma: In the Eye of the Beholder" (Beck, 2004b). What I had discussed in my research was that just like beauty, birth trauma lies in the eye of the beholder.

Sometimes to help illustrate a theme I include an image that one of my participants had sent me along with her narrative. One such example comes from a phenomenological study of mine on subsequent childbirth after a previous birth trauma (Beck & Watson, 2010). A mother sent me a poster of

FIGURE 12.2

Five Essential Themes of PTSD After Childbirth

Theme #		Theme
1	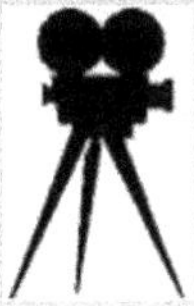	Going to the movies: Please don't make me go!
2	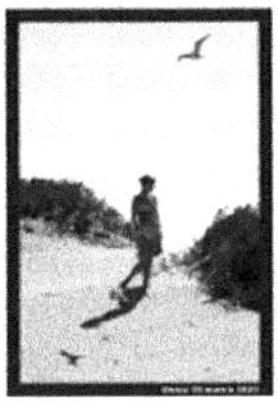	A shadow of myself: Too numb to try and change
3	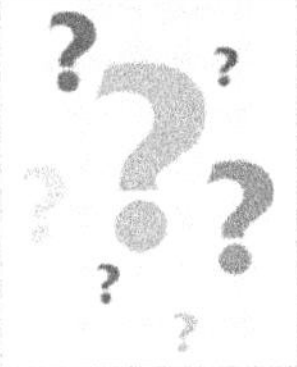	Seeking to have questions answered and wanting to talk, talk, talk
4	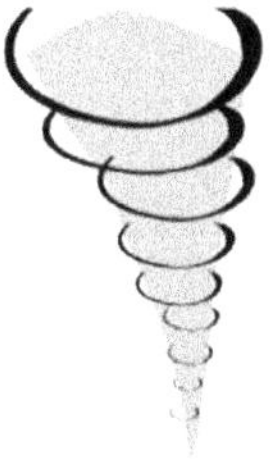	The dangerous trio of anger, anxiety, and depression: Spiraling downward
5	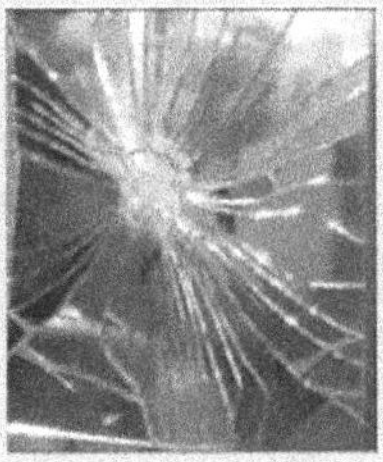	Isolation from the world of motherhood: Dream shattered

Source: Reprinted with permission from Beck, C. T. (2004a). Posttraumatic stress disorder due to childbirth: The aftermath. *Nursing Research, 53*, 216–224. p. 220.

inspirational quotes she hung up in her home (Figure 12.3). This poster helped to bring alive the theme entitled, "Strategizing: Attempts to reclaim their body and complete the journey to motherhood."

FIGURE 12.3

A Poster of Inspirational Quotes by One Mother

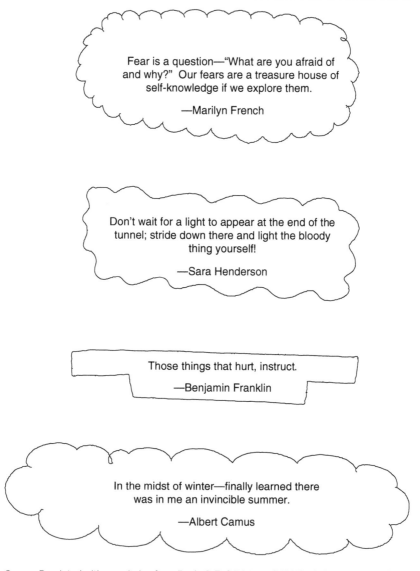

Source: Reprinted with permission from Beck, C. T., & Watson, S.(2010). Subsequent childbirth after a previous traumatic birth, *Nursing Research, 59*, 241–249. p. 246.

FIGURE 12.4

Earthquake Model of Mothers' Posttraumatic Growth After
Birth Trauma

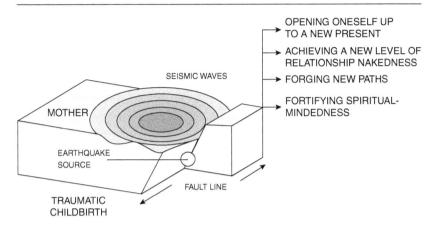

Source: Reprinted with permission from Beck, C. T., & Watson, S.(2016).Posttraumatic growth after birth trauma: "I was broken, now I am unbreakable". *MCN: American Journal of Maternal Child Nursing, 41,* 264–271. p. 268.

The last figure I have included in this chapter comes from my phenomenological study on mothers' posttraumatic growth after birth trauma (Beck & Watson, 2016). In Figure 12.4, I used the metaphor of an earthquake to illustrate the seismic power of traumatic birth that can lead to the four themes of posttraumatic growth. Calhoun and Tedeschi (1998) used the earthquake metaphor in their posttraumatic growth model. They reported that a key to a person developing posttraumatic growth is that a traumatic event shakes the foundation of the individual's assumptive world. This shaking, however, needs to be seismic, just as in an earthquake.

QUALITATIVE REPORTING CHECKLISTS

With the demand for more transparency and rigor in qualitative research, some guidelines for reporting qualitative research have been developed. Two such guidelines are the Consolidated Criteria for Reporting Qualitative Research (COREQ; Tong, Sainsbury, & Craig, 2007) and the Standards for Reporting Qualitative Research (SRQR; O'Brien, Harris, Beckman, Reed, & Cook, 2014). The COREQ guideline consists of a 32-item checklist. One of the limitations of the COREQ is that it addresses only two types of qualitative approaches: interviews and focus groups. The SRQR includes 21 items and was designed to address a wide range of qualitative approaches to assist authors in reporting complete and transparent research. The SRQR, however, does not define methodological rigor. The developers of this guideline therefore stated it would be inappropriate to use it to judge the quality of a study. Qualitative researchers caution that reducing qualitative research to a checklist is too prescriptive and can lead to "the tail wagging the dog," with use of this checklist not conferring methodological rigor (Barbour, 2001).

In summary, this chapter addressed the craft of writing qualitative findings. Strategies for writing a phenomenological study were addressed. Included were examples of figures used in some of my published phenomenological studies to help illustrate some of the creative approaches that can be used to bring to life findings of a phenomenological study. In the following chapter, Chapter 13, the focus switches from conducting a single phenomenological study to developing a program of research using phenomenology.

END OF CHAPTER STUDY ACTIVITIES

Choose a descriptive or interpretive phenomenological study that has recently been published in your discipline. This time focus on the writing of the article and answer these questions:

1. Was the article organized and well-written?

2. Did sections of the article flow logically and smoothly from one section to another?

3. Were sections of the article written in sufficient detail, such as sections on sample and data analysis?

4. Did it seem as if the authors devoted too much space to their findings to the detriment of describing their methodology?

5. In the results section, were quotes included to bring alive the themes? If so, how were the quotes introduced? How were the quotes explained?

6. Were diagrams or figures included to help summarize the findings?

7. Did the title of the article and titles of the themes have sufficient grab to capture your interest?

8. Were any of van Manen's features of phenomenological writing present in the findings section, such as lived thoroughness, nearness, intensification, appeal, and epiphany?

9. Does it seem that the authors protected the confidentiality of their participants when introducing their quotes?

10. Were the authors guilty of one of Thorne and Darbyshire's land mines in qualitative writing?

11. Did the authors state they used one of the qualitative reporting checklists? COREQ? SRQR?

REFERENCES

Barbour, R. S. (2001). Checklists for improving rigour in qualitative research: A case of the tail wagging the dog? *British Medical Journal, 322,* 1115–1117.

Beck, C. T. (2004a). Posttraumatic stress disorder due to childbirth: The aftermath. *Nursing Research, 53,* 216–224.

Beck, C. T. (2004b). Birth trauma: In the eye of the beholder. *Nursing Research, 53,* 28–35.

Beck, C. T., & Watson, S. (2008). Impact of birth trauma on breastfeeding: A tale of two pathways. *Nursing Research, 57,* 228–236.

Beck, C. T., & Watson, S. (2010). Subsequent childbirth after a previous traumatic birth. *Nursing Research, 59,* 241–249.

Beck, C. T., & Watson, S. (2016). Posttraumatic growth after birth trauma: "I was broken, now I am unbreakable." *MCN: American Journal of Maternal Child Nursing, 41,* 264–271.

Calhoun, L. G., & Tedeschi, R. G. (1998). Posttraumatic growth: Future directions. In R. G. Tedeschi, C. L. Park, & L. G. Calhoun (Eds.), *Posttraumatic growth: Positive change in the aftermath of crisis* (pp. 215–238). Mahwah, NJ: Lawrence Erlbaum Associates.

Eisner, E. (1998). *The enlightened eye: Qualitative inquiry and the enhancement of educational practice.* Upper Saddle River, NJ: Merril.

Gadamer, H. G. (1986). *The relevance of the beautiful and other essays.* (N. Walker, Trans.). Cambridge, UK: Cambridge University Press.

Graff, G., & Birkenstein, C. (2018). *They say I say: The moves that matter in academic writing.* New York, NY: W.W. Norton and Company.

Morse, J. M. (2010). "Cherry picking": Writing from thin data. *Qualitative Health Research, 20,* 3.

O'Brien, B. C., Harris, I. B., Beckman, T. J., Reed, D. A., & Cook, D. A. (2014). Standards for reporting qualitative research: A synthesis of recommendations. *Academic Medicine, 89*, 1245–1251.

Richardson, L. (1994). Writing: A method of inquiry. In N. K. Denzin & Y. S. Lincoln (Eds.), *Handbook of qualitative research* (pp. 516–529). Thousand Oaks, CA: SAGE.

Ricoeur, P. (1991). *From text to action: Essays in hermeneutics, II.* (K. Blamey & J. B. Thompson, Trans.). Evanston, IL: Northwestern University Press.

Sandelowski, M. (1994). The use of quotes in qualitative research. *Research in Nursing and Health, 17,* 479–482.

Sandelowski, M. (1998). Writing a good read: Strategies for re-presenting qualitative data. *Research in Nursing & Health, 21,* 375–382.

Thorne, S., & Darbyshire, P. (2005). Land mines in the field: A modest proposal for improving the craft of qualitative health research, *Qualitative Health Research, 15,* 1105–1113.

Tong, A., Sainbury, P., & Craig, J. (2007). Consolidated criteria for reporting qualitative research (COREQ): A 32-item checklist for interviews and focus groups. *International Journal for Quality in Health Care, 19,* 349–357.

van Manen, M. (1990). *Researching lived experience.* New York, NY: State University of New York Press.

van Manen, M. (2014). *Phenomenology of practice.* Walnut Creek, CA: Left Coast Press.

Developing a Program of Research Using Phenomenology

In the introduction to this book I wrote that phenomenology is such a valuable gift to qualitative researchers because it gives us a privileged view of the meaning of endless numbers of experiences from the perspectives of our participants. The focus of this book has been on conducting a single phenomenological study. Here in this chapter I want to provide an example of a program of research using phenomenology and how it provides an enlightening opportunity to walk a mile in the shoes of women who have experienced traumatic childbirth. Phenomenology can skillfully bring visibility to invisible phenomenon for researchers in any discipline. I used five of my phenomenological studies to develop a middle range theory of traumatic childbirth (Beck, 2015).

....

A program of research is "a sustained, systematically planned series of studies addressing a particular gap in the knowledge base of a discipline that is knowledge driven and not method limited" (Beck, 2016, p. 1). A successful research trajectory builds on previous studies and leads to a logical progression of knowledge that fills the identified gap. Eisner (1998) likened the development of a research program to the preparation of a fine meal. He explained that "a model of knowledge accumulation is less like making deposits to a bank account than preparing a fine meal" (p. 211) where each course is connected with and complements the others.

My five studies that I will highlight in this final chapter were all descriptive phenomenological studies using Colaizzi's (1978) methodology (Beck, 2004a, 2004b, 2006; Beck & Watson, 2008; Beck & Watson, 2010). Each study on traumatic childbirth built on the previous study. If phenomenological researchers listen carefully to their participants, oftentimes their participants provide valuable clues to what the researchers' next course in preparing their fine meal should be. For example, in the second study in my research program, I conducted research on posttraumatic stress disorder (PTSD) due to birth trauma (Beck, 2004b). In interviewing one mother about her PTSD, she shared that her

> Child turned 3 years old a few weeks ago. I suppose the pain was not so acute this time. I actually made him a birthday cake and was grateful that I could go to work and not think about the significance of the day. The pain was less, but it was replaced by a numbness that still worries me. I hope that as time passes I can forge some kind of real closeness with this child. I am still unable to tell him I love him but I can now hold him and have times when I am proud of him. I have come a long, long way. (p. 222)

This one paragraph gave me the insight for my next study, which needed to focus on mothers' experiences struggling with the anniversary of their birth trauma, which is always a day of celebration of their child's birthday (Beck, 2006).

In Chapter 12, the creativity needed in writing up a phenomenological study in order for it to have that all-important grab was addressed. In considering the title of my middle range theory, I decided on "The Ever-Widening Ripple Effect" not only for its grab factor but also to convey how just a few minutes or hours in labor and delivery can result in the spreading out of ripples that can have larger, long-term adverse consequences for women (Beck, 2015).

The five phenomenological studies in my research program were as follows in their sequential order:

- Birth trauma in the eye of the beholder (Beck, 2004a)

- Posttraumatic stress disorder due to childbirth: The aftermath (Beck, 2004b)

- The anniversary of birth trauma: Failure to rescue (Beck, 2006)

- Impact of birth trauma on breastfeeding: A tale of two pathways (Beck & Watson, 2008)

- Subsequent childbirth after a previous traumatic birth (Beck & Watson, 2010)

Each course in my meal preparation for research on traumatic childbirth was conducted via the Internet. With the help of Trauma and Birth Stress (TABS; www.tabs.org.nz), a recruitment notice was placed on their website. TABS is a charitable trust located in New Zealand that supports women who have experienced birth trauma. Women were given my e-mail address at the University of Connecticut where they could contact me if they were interested in participating in the research. Women sent me their narratives of their traumatic birth experiences via e-mail.

At first I was leery of using the Internet to collect qualitative data because I would not physically be there with the mothers during their interviews and could not convey my caring to these participants. I was concerned I would not get the rich, thick slices of data I usually had gotten when I interviewed women in person. To my surprise and delight I believe I received richer data because women were able to pick away a little at a time on their stories of birth trauma, saving it on the computer, and coming back to it another day to continue working on it. There was only so much mothers could handle at a time reliving their traumatic births. I believe if I had instead interviewed women in person for about 1 hour, there would have been a limit to what they could share and my data would have been thinner. So from my experiences qualitative researchers should consider obtaining data via the Internet as a possible option.

From these five phenomenological studies, I developed a middle range theory of traumatic childbirth which I entitled "The Ever-Widening Ripple Effect" (Beck, 2015; Figure 13.1). Morse's (2017) method of theoretical coalescence was used where a series of studies on a topic is combined into a whole to create a higher, more abstract middle range theory.

FIGURE 13.1

Traumatic Childbirth: The Ever-Widening Ripple Effect

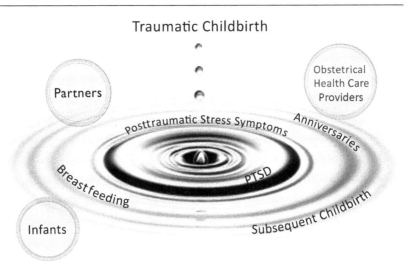

Source: Reprinted with permission from Beck, C. T. (2015). Middle range theory of traumatic childbirth: The ever-widening ripple effect. *Global Qualitative Nursing Research.* doi: 10.1177/2333393615575313.

When a single stone is dropped in a pond it results in ripples spreading out, with each one larger than the previous one. Phenomenology helped reveal what it was about childbirth that women could perceive as traumatic and for some go on to be diagnosed with PTSD and have other long-term consequences. In other words, what did that stone look like that could result in those adverse widening ripples for mothers? So my first study's aim was to discover just that. One mother in that study shared her experience of the event or stone that started the ripples. "I am amazed that 3½ hours in the labor and delivery room could cause such utter destruction in my life. It truly was like being the victim of a violent crime or rape" (Beck, 2004a, p. 32). Using Colaizzi's (1978) method, four themes emerged that described the essence of the experience of traumatic childbirth:

- To care for me: Was that too much to ask for?

- To communicate with me: Why was this neglected?

- To provide safe care: You betrayed my trust, and I felt powerless.

- The end justifies the means: At whose expense? At what price?

What descriptive phenomenology revealed was that women who perceived their births had been traumatic were systematically stripped of protective layers during a time in their lives when they were so vulnerable.

The second phenomenological study focused on the first ripple, that of PTSD, which up to 4.0% of women in community samples and 18.5% in high-risk groups can experience due to birth trauma (Yildiz, Ayers, & Phillips, 2017). Women's description of their experiences yielded five themes:

- Going to the movies: Please don't make me go!

- A shadow of myself: Too numb to try and change

- Seeking to have questions answered and wanting to talk, talk, talk

- A dangerous trio of anger, anxiety, and depression: Spiraling downward

- Isolation from the world of motherhood: Dreams shattered

These themes mirrored the trio of symptoms of PTSD in general: Intrusions, Avoidance, and Arousal. But in this study they were put in the all-important context of new motherhood.

The next phenomenological study in sequential order in my research program focused on the ripple of the impact of birth trauma on women's breastfeeding experiences. Descriptive phenomenology revealed that even though all 52 women in this study perceived their births to have been traumatic, there were two different paths women took. One path promoted breastfeeding, and the other impeded it. Three of the eight themes facilitated breastfeeding: Proving oneself as a mother, Atonement to the infant, and Healing mentally. The other five themes, however, hindered breastfeeding: Intruding flashbacks, Disturbing detachment, Enduring physical pain, Insufficient milk supply, and Feeling violated.

Subsequent childbirth after a previous birth trauma was yet another ripple that, by using descriptive phenomenology, visibility was brought to this long-term consequence of birth trauma. Colaizzi's (1978) method of data analysis yielded four themes:

- Riding the turbulent wave of panic during pregnancy
- Strategizing: Attempts to reclaim their body and complete the journey to motherhood
- Bringing reverence to the birthing process and empowering women
- Still elusive: The longed-for healing birth experience

In the final chapter of this book, Chapter 14, strategies for teaching phenomenological research are presented to help researchers with their responsibility to prepare the next generation of qualitative scholars.

REFERENCES

Beck, C. T. (2004a). Birth trauma: In the eye of the beholder. *Nursing Research*, 53, 28–35.

Beck, C. T. (2004b). Post-traumatic stress disorder due to childbirth: The aftermath. *Nursing Research*, 53, 216–224.

Beck, C. T. (2006). The anniversary of birth trauma: Failure to rescue. *Nursing Research*, 55, 381–390.

Beck, C. T. (2015). Middle range theory of traumatic childbirth: The ever-widening ripple effect. *Global Qualitative Nursing Research*. doi: 10.1177/233339 3615575313

Beck, C. T. (2016). *Developing a program of research in nursing*. New York, NY: Springer Publishing Company.

Beck, C. T., & Watson, S. (2008). Impact of birth trauma on breastfeeding: A tale of two pathways. *Nursing Research*, 57, 228–236.

Beck, C. T., & Watson, S. (2010). Subsequent childbirth after a previous traumatic birth. *Nursing Research, 59,* 241–249.

Colaizzi, P. H. (1978). Psychological research as the phenomenologist views it. In R. S. Valle & M. King (Eds.), *Existential phenomenological alternatives for psychology* (pp. 48–71). New York, NY: Oxford University Press.

Eisner, E. (1998). *The enlightened eye: Qualitative inquiry and the enhancement of educational practice.* Upper Saddle River, NJ: Merril.

Morse, J. M. (2017). *Analyzing and conceptualizing the theoretical foundations of nursing.* New York, NY: Springer Publishing Company.

Yildiz, P. D., Ayers, S., & Phillips, L. (2017). The prevalence of posttraumatic stress disorder in pregnancy and after birth: A systematic review and meta-analysis. *Journal of Affective Disorders, 208,* 634–645.

Teaching Phenomenology

PREPARING OUR NEXT GENERATION OF RESEARCHERS

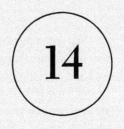

As we prepare the next generation of phenomenological researchers, faculty teaching strategies come into play. First, teaching approaches that other faculty have published are described in this chapter. Following these are examples of my own teaching assignments I use with my PhD students in nursing in my qualitative methodology courses at the University of Connecticut. Ending this chapter is a section on helpful hints for conducting a phenomenological study that I have learned over the years. In the appendix are two proposals of mine. One is for a descriptive phenomenological study entitled "Mothers' Experiences of Posttraumatic Growth Following Traumatic Birth." The second proposal is for an interpretive phenomenological study, "The Lived Experience of the Impact of a Traumatic Birth on Mothers' Caring for their Children." These are included as illustrations for helping students write a proposal for a phenomenological study.

....

OTHER FACULTY MEMBERS' TEACHING STRATEGIES

There is a dearth of published examples of specific approaches to teaching phenomenology. Halling (2012) teaches phenomenology through highlighting experience. Key to his teaching is the pedagogical assumption that theory and practice are inextricably linked characteristics of human life. Halling uses the following analogy that guides his teaching:

> I ask the students who own cars how many of them read the owner's manual to find out how to change a tyre before having a flat; Very few have. Of course the ideal is to practice actually changing a tyre, following the manual, under ideal conditions (good light, enough time, and a dry and comfortable location such as a garage) before one has a flat. (p. 2)

His use of this analogy emphasizes the interconnection of theory and practice and asserts that phenomenology is also a craft. Getting students involved with and reflecting on experience are critical in teaching phenomenology.

Halling (2012) described the teaching approach he uses in an undergraduate level qualitative research methods course. He had students work together in small groups on a small phenomenological topic that the students selected. At the start of the semester, students learned about the dialogue phenomenological approach where researchers start by writing down their own descriptions of the phenomenon under study (Halling, Leifer, & Rowe, 2006). Students then discussed their descriptions in their small groups prior to obtaining a description of the experience from research participants outside of their small group. From students' writing and sharing their own descriptions of the phenomenon under study within their small groups, Halling found that "the phenomenon truly becomes a 'partner' in their research endeavor, or even a 'presence' in the room" (Halling et al., 2006, p. 4). In the dialogal approach, that Halling employed with his class in learning phenomenology through the open discussion of their experiences, the phenomenon took center stage and provided a clear direction for the students. Often themes started to unfold as students listened to each other's experiences. The next challenge for the students was to uncover the core of the experience being studied. This called for moving from the specific to the general.

Another exercise Halling required of his undergraduates involved their becoming familiar with Giorgi's (2009) descriptive phenomenological approach. Again working in small groups Halling provided students with a written description by a woman who experienced religious disillusionment. Students were to use Giorgi's steps to analyze this narrative. Prior to being given this group assignment, the students had previously learned about the necessity of bracketing in descriptive phenomenology. At first students were judgmental about this young woman's becoming disillusioned with religion and her God. As students began to break down her description into meaning units and summarized the psychological meaning in each unit, they began to realize they had been evaluating the woman's experience from their own point of view and not allowing themselves to open up to her perspective. Even though students had read and learned about bracketing, it really had not made an impact on them until they needed to actually practice it. The experiential focus in teaching phenomenology was crucial if students were to really understand phenomenology.

Churchill (2012) stressed that the challenge of teaching phenomenology focuses on professors finding ways of communicating to their students how to embody phenomenology as a process and not just to learn it as a content area. The critical question is "How do we break from the 'first person singular experience' in order to encounter other sentient beings in the world?" (p. 1). His answer is second person perspectivity, which is a mode of resonating with the experiences of others. First and third person perspectives are transcended when students allow themselves to resonate with the other: where the student becomes the "second person" whom the other person addresses.

Regarding this all-important second person perspective in doing phenomenology, Churchill (2012) used creative pedagogical exercises to attune students to this. His exercises helped students become more aware of their ability to experience and understand others' experiences of life. His exercises were aimed at cultivating students' empathetic presence to accessing others' experiences. He described three of these class exercises: going to the cinema, trips to the zoo, and field trips to museums. In watching films, students got a glimpse of what it was like on the other side. Churchill, though, wanted his students to get more attuned to their bodies, so this entailed field trips to zoos or museums. At a local zoo, Churchill asked his students to each choose a particular animal and reflect on its world and compare it to their own personal world. Works of art at a museum were the final example of Churchill's (2012) using lifeworld contexts to aid his students in learning phenomenology. As the students began their field trip, Churchill set the stage by telling them to think of a piece of art as a gesture to them from the artist. His instructions were to

> Just let the artwork select you, rather than the other way around. Trust the fact that you were compelled to do a double-take when you just walked past it, and try to notice the kind of dance you do with it, finding just the right vantage point from which to observe it. When you find that point, try to notice how you felt, how you are affected in that very place. (p. 5)

By his class exercises at the zoo, cinema, or museum, Churchill provided students the opportunity to practice second person perspectivity through their embodied encounters with others as they became attuned to what was revealed to them when they interacted with the other. As students moved to the second person experience, there was a shift from being enveloped in oneself to a centering on the communication and gestures of the other, and a deeper encounter was possible.

In Hultgren's (1995) graduate course in phenomenological inquiry, she stressed to her students that it is only by doing phenomenology that they can really understand it. She recalled Heidegger's (1971) words, "We shall never learn what is called swimming, for example, or what it calls for by reading a treatise on swimming. Only the leap into the river tells us what is called swimming" (p. 20). She designed her course to provide such a leap for her students to guide them in learning what phenomenology is.

MY TEACHING STRATEGIES

Now in this latter half of the chapter my own teaching assignments are described. "Teaching phenomenology demands a suspension of existing dogmas by orienting to primary sources, scholarly phenomenological traditions, exemplary practices, and leading authors" (Adams & van Manen, 2017, p. 780). I definitely support the need for PhD students to read the primary sources of the different descriptive and interpretive phenomenological methods in order to prevent method slurring. My students read the primary sources of Colaizzi (1978); Giorgi (2009); van Kaam (1966); Dahlberg, Dahlberg, and Nyström (2008); van Manen (1990); Benner (1994); and Smith, Flowers, and Larkin (2009) in regard to each of their phenomenological methodologies. First, however, before reading on specific methods, I have my students read the primary sources of Husserl and Heidegger so they understand the philosophical underpinnings that distinguish descriptive from interpretive phenomenology.

Merleau-Ponty (1962) stressed that the doing of phenomenology is the way one can really understand it. I support his assertion, and that is why I have each of my students conduct their own descriptive phenomenological pilot study. I teach a core course entitled Introduction to Qualitative Methodology to the PhD students in nursing at the University of Connecticut. There is a semester-long project for this course that consists of each student independently conducting a descriptive phenomenological pilot study using Colaizzi's (1978) method. Each student chooses a phenomenon to study related to their dissertation topic. The first part of this assignment is to develop a proposal for their descriptive phenomenological pilot study of their chosen phenomenon. The phenomenological research proposal outline I use as the guide is located in Table 14.1. Once I approve their proposals, each doctoral student recruits a purposive sample of three individuals who have experienced the phenomenon they are studying. After obtaining informed consent, interviews are audiotaped and subsequently transcribed by the students. Data generated from their interviews are analyzed using Colaizzi's method. Findings are then written up, and a final paper is submitted the last day of class. Each week during the second half of the class students share their progress to date on their pilot studies. As Eisner (1998) stated, "Nothing replaces being there. Being there means that novice researchers can talk to the teacher and to the other students about their work, their aims, their satisfactions, and their frustrations" (p. 233).

During each class, I guide students through Colaizzi's step-by-step data analysis process. In Table 14.2 is an exercise I use to introduce my students to the beginning steps of Colaizzi's method. It is an excerpt from an interview I

TABLE 14.1

Outline for a Proposal for a Phenomenological Research Study

I. Introduction
- Phenomenon of interest
- Brief background of the problem
- Statement of the problem
- Purpose of the study
- Significance of the study for your discipline

II. Review of the Literature
- Search strategy and results
- Synthesize relevant literature
- Critically evaluate pertinent research
- Identify gaps in knowledge your study will fill

III. Methodology
- Research questions
- Research design (descriptive or interpretive phenomenology)
- Philosophical underpinnings
- Population and sample (selection, sample size, inclusion criteria)
- Setting
- Researcher's perspective (for epoché and reduction)
- Data collection (interview technique, audiotaping, field notes, etc.)
- Ethical considerations (informal consent plus process consent)
- Data analysis (specific method, e.g., van Manen, Colaizzi, qualitative software)
- Limitations

IV. Anticipated Timetable

V. Budget

VI. References

VII. Appendices (consent form, supporting documents, participant profile sheet)

conducted with a mother suffering with postpartum depression. I have the students read it over and highlight significant statements. Next I have them identify some repeated potential themes that already are present in just a portion of this interview. There purposely is a wide margin on the right side so that there is room for the students to write the repetitive phrases they have identified. I give the students the excerpt of the interview that neither has those significant statements underlined nor the potential themes labeled on the right side. I just included both of those in the table so you have the complete example. Once students have finished, we go over what repetitive patterns they identified already in just a portion

TABLE 14.2

Excerpt From Postpartum Depression Interview

Res: Well, it's very <u>scary.</u> You feel as though you are <u>not the same person</u>, that you are <u>afraid</u> that your children aren't going to have you for a mother. You are <u>afraid</u> ah, I married a very good, a very supportive husband and very supportive the whole time, and yet I married a very positive, you know, a very perceptive person, and here I was. I was extremely <u>insecure</u>. I was <u>scared to be left alone</u>. I <u>cried</u> all the time. I, you know, you start thinking, what kind of a wife am I? How can he come home to this, you know, how am I going to have a happy marriage? I mean, like you feel so good, but I'm so, so out of control and, and I, I thought that even if I got better, which I, my big <u>fear</u> was that <u>I wasn't going to get better</u>, and also that I was going to be labeled something that, that I wasn't, that. I had another feeling, even if I got better that I wasn't, still <u>wasn't going to be the person I was,</u> before the experience. That I never would quite get over it. And ah, I, I know, I thought about how would I be if I kept coming home and, and he was a mess all the time. I mean, eventually I would get fed up with it, you know. And so I didn't, I couldn't relax, I had a lot of <u>anxiety</u> [unintelligible—over the reports ??] that it was going to take time to get better. I mean, people were telling me, "Oh, yeah, you know it's been a year and I feel stronger, you know, every week I feel a little stronger." I'm going, "A year, I couldn't live a year with a man that was going through this." You know, and so you feel like your whole world is falling apart.	Scary Not same person Afraid Insecure Scared, Cried Fear Not going to get better Wasn't going to be person I was Anxiety

Your kids aren't going to have the life you wanted them to have, and everything. Some of the <u>questions</u> that I definitely wanted answered for me is, if it was possible to be cured and not just on permanent treatment, was I, you know, if, if the people that had gone through this were actually cured. If I was going to meet a bunch of people that were on permanent therapy and, and had that to look forward to, or if, I wanted to know I was going to better. These were <u>questions</u> I had to ask somebody, if, if they were cured, how I described, how did you feel and how were you treated? You know, by the doctor and everything, what did, what was the treatment? What did therapy involve? Was it just medication? What were they doing, and how was it helping her? I wanted to know how normal she was now, how really normal, obviously, she, she was now. And I, I wanted a lot of <u>reinforcement that I was going to be well.</u> That I was going to be, not just well, that I <u>was going to be normal again</u>, back the way I was. How, ah, sometimes also I would feel completely okay, only to have, totally without notice, just a feeling overcame. I could feel it come physically on me. And like, pull me out of, like I'd be ah, having guests or family over for dinner and laughing and talking and it was just like, pulled my personality right out of me and I'd just be quiet and looking around, and, and <u>start acting</u> again, and just the minute before I was normal. So feeling normal didn't really comfort me, because it would come and go, come and go. So I was going to ask <u>questions</u> like if they had that problem even after so many years.	Questions Questions Reinforcement that would be normal again Acting Questions

(Continued)

TABLE 14.2 (Continued)

When she was sitting there telling me that she was normal, does she have reoccurrences still being treated? And these are the feelings. I had to write this down, because when I felt normal it seemed like that really <u>wasn't real</u>, and then it would come back and, and I would feel like it was never going to go away.	Felt I wasn't real
I felt extremely <u>anxious.</u> Like a cat. And, that's totally ah, contrary to my usual nature. I'm a very laid back person. I felt	Anxious
<u>alienated</u> and <u>isolated.</u> I <u>never wanted to be alone</u>. I, I <u>didn't feel a bond with anybody.</u> I, I, ah, even when I was with people I felt <u>withdrawn</u>. People were telling me, I was very quiet, and that was the opposite. I'm a very outgoing person. I like people. I felt depressed and, and totally <u>insecure. Insecure</u> was a big feeling. I, I felt	Isolated Didn't feel bond with anybody Withdrawn
like that I needed all the help I could get and, and that made me <u>insecure</u> because I'm used to being independent and you don't like the feeling of dependency. And also, that you also keep thinking it, about	Insecure
your marriage. I, I mean, you're <u>insecure,</u> so you're <u>insecure</u> in your marriage but you're also <u>insecure,</u> thinking, my husband didn't marry an <u>insecure</u> woman. He was attracted to how confident, and what I was before. He wouldn't have married someone	Insecure
that was <u>insecure</u> and <u>crying</u> all the time. All the things I was proud about in myself are gone. You know, I'm a basket case.	Insecure
And most, I was very <u>scared</u>, like I said, that I wasn't going to be a good mother,	Scared
a good wife, and that I was <u>never going to be happy again.</u> But I never, I didn't any choice.	Never be happy again

I had <u>fear, anxiety</u>, and , and feelings like that, so it's like <u>no joy</u>, you know when I look at, the new baby I would think he was a beautiful baby, and I'd try to focus on that because I love children. But that real deep <u>joy that you have wasn't there</u>.	fear/anxiety No joy Deep joy wasn't there
Res: [<u>Crying</u> as she speaks] Yeah, but, I feel like they've stole that time from me. When you take home your new baby, that I, even when I had depression, after the other two, that I still [unintelligible] the kind of depression when you know it's all your fault, because the baby's so perfect and you want to be a perfect mother and you ah, you become very aware of your faults and things. But this was completely different. It was like a <u>withdrawal of emotions.</u> I, I <u>didn't even feel real</u>. Mostly, I can say, I <u>didn't feel real</u>. I felt like I was <u>acting</u>. It was like, someone gave me something horrible like, drugs. I went through the motions of my life <u>without any of the joy</u>. I didn't, everything seemed futile. Why I'd do this, why bother doing that. There was no, nothing I have enjoyed doing. And ah, nothing I looked forward to and ah, the only feelings I had were <u>anxiety</u>, and <u>fear</u>, and <u>isolation</u>. And ah, what's wrong, and things like that. I, I didn't laugh naturally, you know, and I didn't have any of those kind of feelings, or the other feelings were so intense. I <u>don't know if positive feelings were ever present</u>. So, ah, mostly, this is mostly I was <u>scared</u>. I was <u>afraid</u> I wouldn't get better. I was <u>afraid</u> they were going to just give me a label, like, like I was never normal. That, and then, that I'd be on treatment the rest of my life.	Crying Withdrawal of emotions Didn't feel real Acting Without any joy Anxiety Fear, Isolation Lack of positive feelings Scared Afraid

(Continued)

TABLE 14.2 (Continued)

The treatment would make me act normal, but it wouldn't make me normal. And ah, or they'd give me the wrong treatment, that, which would aggravate my condition and that gave me a big fear cause I already couldn't stand the way I was. And if they gave me something that aggravated it that I, I, I was very <u>afraid</u> ah, they would aggravate my condition trying to treat me. You know as well as I do being in the medical field that's a big possibility. I was very <u>afraid</u> I wouldn't be well to raise my children. They wouldn't have me, for what, how I know myself for a mother and that's what I wanted them to have, because you don't want your children just in good hands. You want your fingerprints on their lives.	Afraid Afraid

of one interview. Some of these repetitive patterns include the mother feeling scared, no joy, afraid, anxious, isolated, not real, like she is acting, and insecure.

Students sometimes have difficulty writing formulated meanings of the significant statements they have extracted from their interviews for their pilot studies. In Table 14.3 is an example of another exercise I have the students do in class. The significant statements are from a phenomenological study I have conducted on the anniversary of traumatic childbirth (Beck, 2006). I have provided the answers for the actual formulated meanings here in the right column of this table so that you can have a complete exercise with answers included. I ask the students to read over the significant statements in the left column and write their corresponding formulated meanings in the right column. Once they finish writing these formulated meanings, we go over them in class to provide guidance in this challenging step of Colaizzi's (1978) method. What I find students doing initially is not staying close to the words the participant said. Students are interpreting, which they should not be doing in a descriptive phenomenological study. For example, if the participant said she was worried about something, in the formulated meaning the student would not use the word, "worried" but would say the person "was afraid." Being worried is not the same as being afraid.

My rationale for having my PhD students interview only three participants is due to the time limitation in one semester. I want to be able to guide them from start to finish with their pilot study. If they were to continue to collect data until saturation, they could never have finished the project by the end

TABLE 14.3

Formulated Meaning Exercise With Answers for Anniversary of Birth Trauma

Significant statements	Formulated meanings
A. "I felt full of rage at the selfish people who stole the birth of my son from me and now manage to steal the fun of his birthday from me each year."	The mother felt full of rage at the selfish clinicians who stole not only her son's birth from her but also the fun of his birthday for her each year.
B. "My self-esteem was really low that day. I felt like a complete failure as a mother."	The mother's self-esteem was really low on the day of the anniversary of her traumatic birth leaving her feeling like a complete failure as a mother.
C. "I felt overwhelmed with sadness and grief over what I had to endure that day.	The mother felt overwhelmed with sadness and grief over what she had endured during the day of her traumatic birth.
D. "I felt such guilt because I wasn't truly 'there'—mind, body, or spirit on her birthday."	The mother felt such guilt because she felt she wasn't truly present in mind, body, or spirit on her daughter's birthday.
E. "I was angry when my family and friends didn't mention the birth or my hospital experience at all.	The mother was angry on the day of her daughter's birthday when neither her family nor friends did not mention her birth or her hospital experience.

of the semester. After the qualitative course is over, some doctoral students go on to continue their pilot studies to data saturation. Many students have used their pilot data to present posters at research presentations, and some go on to use their pilot studies as the basis for their dissertations. Below are the reflections of one of my former PhD students' experiences, Carrie Morgan Eaton (2018), in conducting this descriptive phenomenological pilot study as part of her course work for my introductory qualitative research course:

> I had the opportunity to conduct a pilot study in my first qualitative research course with Dr. Beck during my PhD program at the University

of Connecticut School of Nursing. The title of my pilot study was "The Experiences of Recovered Anorexic Mothers Feeding Their Children." Dr. Beck introduced me to Colaizzi's (1978) descriptive phenomenology during my initial semester of coursework. This was my first experience immersing myself into an Institutional Review Board approved research study. Embarking on constructing a proposal into a feasible pilot research project initially seemed like a daunting task. Refining my ideas into a tangible research project in the timeline of one semester was a challenge. Each week our PhD cohort shared the status of his or her progress. This weekly practice not only provided an arena of constructive feedback and encouragement, but it also offered a level of accountability. Articulating the details of my research study to my peers forced me to engage in scholarly dialogue and was extremely beneficial to my confidence as a researcher. Under Dr. Beck's exceptional guidance along with the support of my colleagues in the PhD cohort, I successfully conducted my first research study. Following Colaizzi's (1978) method of descriptive phenomenology, I audiotaped three face-to-face interviews and transcribed them verbatim. I had a strict one-semester timeline in completing my pilot research and had to remain focused. Following transcription I analyzed the data receiving weekly feedback from Dr. Beck and my colleagues in class to craft my work carefully. The result was a completed pilot study. I successfully conveyed the results of my research into both a paper and a poster presentation which I presented at national conferences. This provided me with a sense of accomplishment in looking to the future.

Over the course of the first semester in the doctoral program, I had the opportunity to access NVivo, a qualitative data analysis (QDA) package that was free of charge to university students and faculty. I deliberately chose to analyze my data via the systematic, iterative process taught by Dr. Beck followed by a comparison of the process using qualitative data analysis software. I was able to compare the two methods and guide my decision toward a future preference of qualitative data analysis software.

After presenting the outcome of my pilot study at a nursing conference, I was asked to consider publishing the results. While I had the full support of Dr. Beck to move forward, I felt the data were not saturated yet. After careful consideration and consultation with Dr. Beck, I decided my dissertation would focus on carrying out the pilot study I started during my first semester of the PhD program. Expanding on my pilot study allowed me to surpass my initial goal of 10 participants to a purposeful sample of 16 mothers who self-identified as recovered from anorexia nervosa. Building on my pilot work secured the confidence I needed to achieve my goal of a completed dissertation.

In closing, capturing the essentials of collection, analysis, and management of qualitative data for a pilot qualitative research study during my first semester of PhD coursework helped me develop a realistic sense of the scholarly process. Completing a pilot study early in the program focused my intellectual curiosity on my dissertation topic and prepared me to articulate my research interests in a concise manner. Some of the lessons I've learned in conducting research fall back on the first practices Dr. Beck taught me through the pilot study project-including daily reading and writing, adhering to timelines, and accepting constructive feedback. I often reflect with my PhD colleagues on the value of Dr. Beck's qualitative pilot study process as the defining moment that instilled a mental shift from graduate student to capable researcher. (Eaton, 2018)

PhD students from other schools at University of Connecticut are welcome to enroll in my qualitative courses. Students from Business, Public Health, Family Studies, Sports Management, Education, and Communication have energized my seminars over the years. Here are some examples of the breadth of phenomena my students have studied in their pilot work:

- Looking at metastatic cancer from a man's perspective

- Nurses' experiences of symptom management among patients with heart failure

- Teachers' experiences with low socioeconomic status

  students' participation in structured physical activity programming

- Experience of a person having to sell their family business

- Experience of a current or previous eating disorder during pregnancy

- Undergraduate nursing students' experiences communicating with psychiatric patients in mental health settings

- Experiences of nurses serving on interprofessional health care governing boards

- Nurses' experiences in supporting parents to hold their infants skin to skin

- Experiences of female executives returning to the workplace after childbirth

- Members' experiences in team conflict

- Experiences of lifestyle changes among Middle Eastern graduate students in the United States

- Experiences of volunteers in Haiti regarding sexual health of adolescents

- Communicating science with the public: A meteorology perspective

- Experience of adopting a child with special needs

- Experiences of young African American women who participated in an adolescent pregnancy prevention program

PHENOMENOLOGY TIPS

From my years both conducting phenomenological studies and teaching PhD students qualitative research methodologies, I have compiled a number of helpful hints I would like to share.

- No matter which specific phenomenological research design you choose to use, you need to always read the primary sources of that methodology. So for instance if you choose to conduct an interpretive phenomenological design using van Manen's approach, then you should read all the books and articles published by van Manen to help guide you in correctly using his approach. You never want to be guilty of method slurring.

- Reading primary sources also goes for the underlying philosophy of your chosen phenomenological design. So if you decide to conduct a descriptive phenomenological study, you need to read books written by Husserl so you have an in-depth understanding of his philosophy that will guide your research.

- It is difficult to know in advance the sample size you will need to reach data saturation. When your participants describe their experiences only in generalities without many specific examples, you will need more participants than anticipated. If, however, your participants describe their experiences in depth with many specific examples of points they are making, you will need fewer participants in your sample.

- When I am setting up the time and place for the interviews, I tell my participants how I will begin the interview so they can prepare and think about their experiences. I tell them that any specific examples that they can share at the time of the interview will be extremely valuable.

- Before I start an interview I explain to my participants that while they are speaking they may see me jot down a word or a phrase. I explain that it is not that they said something wrong. It is just a reminder to me to ask them a follow-up question on that point once the interview is completed.

- Here is the way I start off my phenomenological interviews: "Please share with me your experiences with ____. Describe all your thoughts, feelings, and perceptions about your experience until you have no more to say. Any specific examples of points that you are making will be extremely valuable."

- If you are using a tape recorder, you may be tempted periodically to look at it to make sure it is still recording. Try not to do this because participants will notice your glance and this will remind the participant they are being tape-recorded.

- Often once you turn your smartphone or the tape recorder off the participant will start to say something really important about their experience. Ask the participant if you have their permission to start the recording again.

- During an interview if your participants are describing their experiences only in generalities here is one approach, depending on the phenomenon you are studying, that can be helpful. Ask your participants to choose one day that would best describe the experience being studied. Then ask them to please concentrate on describing that one day in particular from the time they woke up in the morning until the time they went to bed at night. This directs them to speaking on a more specific level. In my research with postpartum depression, this strategy was appropriate since the phenomenon I was studying can occur all day long.

- If participants describe a specific example illustrating a point they were making, give them positive feedback. Then you can ask them if they could provide another example.

- Sometimes participants will provide only a brief, general description of their experiences. Even though this will not be very helpful to you, I always thank participants for sharing their experiences. I tell them what they have shared will be valuable to me in my research.

- I do not interrupt participants during an interview to ask a follow-up question. Only when they are finished speaking do I question them. I am afraid that if I interrupt them in the middle of their interview, what they were going to talk about next, they will not get back to since I would have interrupted their thought process.

- As an ethical practice, once an interview is over I always ask the participants if there was anything they had shared with me during the interview that now they wish they hadn't. If so, I would delete that section from the audiotape before it is transcribed. This is how I practiced consent process with my participants.

- Even though you are audiotaping the interview, it is very helpful to also keep a journal describing what went on during the interview. This can include your emotions during the interview or your reaction to the participant. Nonverbal behaviors of the participant are also important to include. This way when you have transcribed the interview, you can insert the participant's nonverbal communication at the appropriate point in the transcript. For example, if a mother's eyes began to well up with tears when she said something about her experience with postpartum depression, I would note this in my journal and then add it in the appropriate place in the transcript.

- As soon as you can after an interview is completed, write in your journal so you don't forget anything about the interview that you want to make note of. Most of the time when I am interviewing women regarding postpartum depression they want to be interviewed in their homes so they don't have to get a babysitter for their infants. Sometimes after I drive away from their home, I will pull over in a parking lot and jot down a few points I want to make sure I won't forget.

- Interviews conducted in a participant's home at times can be challenging, especially if there are small children in the home. The toddlers may want to keep trying to get to your tape recorder or smartphone if you are using that to record the interview. One strategy I often use is to bring a couple of children's books with me to the interview. While the mother is being interviewed, I have the toddlers sitting on my lap, and I just keep turning the pages of the book to distract them from trying to get to the smartphone or tape recorder.

- Regarding transcriptionists, if your research study focuses on a difficult or sensitive topic, you need to caution and prepare your transcriptionists for what they are about to hear.

- You need to provide your transcriptionists with specific guidelines to follow. For example, if the transcriptionists cannot understand a word or phrase, what do you want them to do? Leave a blank space, highlight the word or phrase in question, or another option.

- Make sure you have a clear agreement with your transcriptionists if you will be paying them by the page. What size font will they use? Will it be double or single spacing? What size will the margins be?

- When researchers use their smartphones to record interviews, this requires special precautions to ensure the security of the interviews. There are special cell phone apps that can encrypt the interview data. Without special encryption, the interviews should be transferred from a cell phone to a secure device as soon as possible and deleted from the cell phone.

- If you are conducting your phenomenological study via e-mail, make sure you take time to individually craft your e-mail response to your participants to make them feel valued.

- As you are analyzing your data, if there is a particularly powerful quote that you think you will include in a manuscript you will write for publication to bring a theme to life, have some way of flagging those quotes. This way when you go to write up your manuscript, it will be easy for you to find these powerful quotes to illustrate your themes.

- If you are conducting your phenomenological study over the Internet, the great benefit is that the interview is already typed and all you have to do is press the print button. If, however, you are conducting a face-to-face interview and audiotaping it, once the interview is transcribed, you need to listen to the tape-recording while you read the transcript to correct any errors the transcriptionist may have made or to fill in the blanks where the transcriptionist was not able to understand what the participant was saying.

- Researchers can use qualitative software to assist in managing all their data. If you do choose this route, please remember that a computer does not have a brain. The computer can organize your data but not analyze it.

- Using or not using qualitative software to assist in managing your data is the choice of the researcher. Qualitative researchers usually feel strongly one way or the other. I prefer not to use qualitative software. I have tried it, and it seems to put up barriers between me as the researcher and my ability to analyze the data.

- Analyzing your data for themes is a time-consuming and iterative process. You often start with a large number of possible themes. As you keep revisiting your analysis, some of the themes you will come to realize should be combined together while others may need to be divided into multiple themes.

In ending, I would like to leave faculty with a quote from Carse (1994):

> We know we have met a teacher when we come away amazed not at what the teacher was thinking, but at what we are thinking. We will forget what the teacher is saying because we are listening to a source deeper than the teachings themselves. A great teacher exposes the source and then steps back. (p. 70)

REFERENCES

Adams, C., & van Manen, M. A. (2017). Teaching phenomenological research and writing. *Qualitative Health Research, 27*, 780–791.

Beck, C. T. (2006). The anniversary of birth trauma: Failure to rescue. *Nursing Research, 55*, 381–390.

Benner, P. (Ed.) (1994). *Interpretive phenomenology: Embodiment, caring, and ethics in health and illness.* Thousand Oaks, CA: SAGE.

Carse, J. P. (1994). *Breakfast at the victory: The mysticism of ordinary experience.* New York, NY: HarperCollins Publishers.

Churchill, S. D. (2012). Teaching phenomenology by way of "second-person perspectivity" (from my thirty years at the University of Dallas). *The Indo-Pacific Journal of Phenomenology, 12,* sup 3, 1–14. doi: 10.2989/IPJP.2012.12.3.6.1114

Colaizzi, P. F. (1978). Psychological research as the phenomenologist views it. In R. Valle & M. King (Eds.), *Existential phenomenological alternative for psychology* (pp. 48–71). New York, NY: Oxford University Press.

Dahlberg, K., Dahlberg, H., & Nyström, M. (2008). *Reflective lifeworld research.* Lund, Sweden: Studentlitteratur.

Eaton, C. M. (2018). *The experiences of recovered anorexic mothers feeding their children.* Unpublished dissertation. Storrs, CT: University of Connecticut.

Eisner, E. W. (1998). *The enlightened eye: Qualitative inquiry and the enhancement of educational practice.* Upper Saddle River, NJ: Prentice-Hall, Inc.

Giorgi, A. (2009). *The descriptive phenomenological method in Psychology: A modified Husserlian approach.* Pittsburgh, PA: Duquesne University Press.

Halling, S. (2012). Teaching phenomenology through highlighting experiences. *Indo-Pacific Journal of Phenomenology, 12*, 6 pp. doi: 10.2989/IPJP.2012.12.3.5.113

Halling, S., Leifer, M., & Rowe, J. O. (2006). The emergence of the dialogal approach: Forgiving another. In C. T. Fischer (Ed.), *Qualitative research methods for psychologists: Introduction through empirical studies* (pp. 173–212). New York, NY: Academic Press.

Heidegger, M. (1971). *On the way to language*. New York, NY: Harper & Row.

Hultgren, F. H. (1995). The phenomenology of "doing" phenomenology: The experience of teaching and learning together. *Human Studies, 18*, 371–388.

Merleau-Ponty, M. (1962). *Phenomenology of perception*. (C. Smith, Trans.). New York, NY: Routledge & Kegan Paul Ltd.

Smith, J. A., Flowers, P., & Larkin, M. (2009). *Interpretative phenomenological analysis*. Los Angeles, CA: SAGE.

van Kaam, A. (1966). *Existential foundations of psychology*. Pittsburgh, PA: Duquesne University Press.

van Manen, M. (1990). *Researching lived experience: Human science for an action sensitive pedagogy*. New York, NY: State University of New York Press.

Glossary

Abstraction. In Smith's interpretive phenomenological analysis, this action involves clustering like with like in a superordinate theme and giving it a name.

Authenticity. The degree to which qualitative researchers are faithful and fair in reporting the range of different perspectives shared by the participants.

Being-in-the-world. This is a Heideggerian term that refers to the manner in which human beings are involved in the world.

Bracketing. In a phenomenological study, the researcher's process of identifying and holding aside his or her preconceived beliefs when collecting and analyzing data.

Bridling. Dahlberg's term for bracketing where reflective lifeworld researchers reflect on their own lifeworld so it does not go unnoticed in the research process.

Composite structural description. The step in Moustakas's modification where the researcher using the composite textural description develops a synthesized structural description that represents the group of participants as a whole.

Composite textural description. In Moustakas's modification, this is the step where the researcher, using the total group of individual textural descriptions, develops a synthesized description.

Confirmability. When evaluating the trustworthiness of a qualitative study, this criterion refers to the objectivity or neutrality of the data and interpretation.

Congruence. The evaluation criterion that addresses whether the process and findings fit together in a qualitative study.

Constituent. A part that takes into account the role or position in the whole.

Contextualization. The step in Smith's interpretive phenomenological analysis where the researcher examines connections among emergent themes by identifying the contextual elements such as temporal or cultural themes.

Corporeality. The fundamental lifeworld theme for van Manen that focuses on the fact persons are always bodily in the world.

Creativity. In assessing a qualitative study, this is the criterion that addresses whether the data have been analyzed, organized, and presented in imaginative ways.

Credibility. In evaluating qualitative studies, this refers to the confidence one has in the truth of the data and findings.

Criticality. In evaluating a qualitative study, this aspect looks at whether the research process demonstrates evidence of critical appraisal.

Dasein. This a Heideggerian term that refers to human beings' ability to wonder about their own being and existence.

Data saturation. In a qualitative study, this is the point where any new data collected are redundant to what already has been found.

Debriefing. Researchers' communication with persons about their experience participating in the research once they have completed the study.

Dependability. In evaluating a qualitative study, this refers to how stable the data are over time and over conditions.

Detailed approach. van Manen's approach to isolating thematic aspects where the researcher looks at every sentence to see what it reveals about the phenomenon under study.

Element. A part is independent of the whole description where it resides.

Epiphany. The dimension of phenomenological writing that provides a transforming effect on readers where they suddenly grasp the meaning of the experience and it stirs them to the core of their being.

Epistemology. A branch of philosophy that examines knowledge and how we come to know about the world as we experience it.

Epoché. This is a Greek word meaning abstention. Husserl used this term to capture the actions a person needs in order to suspend their natural attitude of taken-for-granted beliefs.

Essence. This term refers to that which makes a thing what it is and without it, it would not be what it is.

Essential themes. For van Manen these are themes that are unique to the experience under study.

Exemplars. In Benner's method, these are aspects of a paradigm case or a thematic analysis.

Exhaustive description. In Colaizzi's method, this step is where the researcher integrates all the results of the topic being investigated.

Explication. A term used by van Kaam in regard to the process of making components of a phenomenon explicit that were implicitly experienced in awareness by the participants.

Explicitness. The criterion in assessing a qualitative study that examines whether the methodological decisions, interpretations, and researcher's biases have been addressed.

Formulated meanings. In Colaizzi's method, this is the step where the researcher takes a precarious leap from what participants said to what they mean.

Free imaginative variation. For Husserl, this action helps to discover the essence of a phenomenon. A person mentally removes an aspect of the phenomenon under study in order to determine if its removal radically transforms the description of the phenomenon in an essential way.

Function. The step in Smith's interpretive phenomenological analysis where the researcher examines the emergent themes for their particular function within the transcript.

Fundamental structure. In his method, Colaizzi calls for formulating the exhaustive description in as unequivocal a statement of identification as possible.

Gem. According to Smith, it is a single utterance shared by a participant that has great resonance across the case and corpus.

General structure of a phenomenon. The step in Giorgi's method where the key constituents and the relationship among them are written to identify the essence of the phenomenon as a holistic perspective.

Hermeneutic circle. In conducting a hermeneutic study, the researcher's process of continually moving between the parts and the whole of the text being analyzed and interpreted.

Hermeneutic spiral. The term that Dahlberg prefers to hermeneutic circle. Instead of a circle, she uses a spiral to describe the process because a spiral is open at the beginning as well as at the end.

Horizontalization. In Moustakas's modification, this is the listing of every expression relevant to the experience being studied.

Hypothetical identification. In van Kaam's method, an initial description of the phenomenon under study is written based on his earlier steps of grouping data into categories, reducing vague expressions into more precise descriptive terms.

Incidental themes. In van Manen's method, these themes are incidentally related to the phenomenon or experience being studied and are not essential.

Individual structural description. The step in Moustakas's modification where for each participant the researcher constructs a description of the experience based on the individual textural description and imaginative variation.

Individual textural description. In Moustakas's modification of van Kaam's approach, this description is constructed from the themes and invariant constituents for each participant's experience.

Inquiry audit. This process involves having an external reviewer carefully review all of the documents, data, and audit trail in a qualitative study.

Integrity. This criterion in assessing a qualitative study looks at whether the research reflects repetitive checks of validity and a humble presentation of findings.

Intensification. This refers to the qualitative researcher's use of key words to allow meaning of the experience to come through.

Intentionality. A term used by Husserl indicating the inseparable connectedness of human beings to the world. It is a property of consciousness where humans are always conscious of an object or event, to the experience of the world.

Invariant constituents. In Moustakas's modification of van Kaam's approach, these are the unique qualities of the experience being studied that stand out.

Lived experience. It is a reflexive or self-given awareness of life as we live through it.

Lived thoroughness. This refers to a text that vividly brings an experience to life for the reader.

Meaning units. For Giorgi, meaning units are divisions in an interview transcript where a significant shift in meaning occurs.

Member checking. After analyzing the data, qualitative researchers can return to participants with a draft of the findings to allow them the opportunity to review and comment.

Natural attitude. The everyday ordinary way a person perceives things.

Necessary constituent. For van Kaam, this is a moment of an experience that can be explicitly or implicitly expressed in the significant majority of the participants' descriptions of an experience while also compatible with descriptions that do not include it.

Negative case analysis. Qualitative researchers search for the inclusion of cases that seem to disconfirm earlier findings or interpretations.

Numeration. The step in Smith's method where the researcher makes a frequency count regarding how often an emergent theme is supported.

Ontology. The branch of philosophy that is concerned with Being, what it means to be.

Paradigm case. In Benner's interpretive phenomenological method, this refers to a strong example of the phenomenon under study.

Peer debriefing. This refers to sessions a researcher has with peers to review the findings of their qualitative study.

Persistent observation. During data collection, a qualitative researcher's intense focus on relevant aspects of the phenomenon under study.

Polarization. In Smith's method, this steps includes exploring for oppositional relationships among emergent themes.

Prolonged engagement. A sufficient amount of time a researcher collects data for in order to have in-depth understanding of the group being studied.

Reduction. This term means to lead back. The epoché, by way of bracketing presumptions, is the means of achieving reduction. For Husserl, reduction leads to an attentive turning to the world with an open state of mind.

Relationality. A fundamental lifeworld theme suggested by van Manen that focuses on the relationship persons maintain with other persons.

Selective approach. van Manen's approach to identifying themes where the researcher circles, underlines, or highlights phrases or statements that reveal something about the phenomenon or experience being studied.

Sensitivity. This criterion evaluates whether the qualitative research has been conducted in ways that are sensitive to the nature of human, cultural, and social contexts.

Significant statements. This is the step in Colaizzi's method that entails extracting from transcribed interviews phrases or sentences that directly pertain to the phenomenon being studied.

Spatiality. A fundamental lifeworld theme that refers to filled space.

Subordinate theme. In Smith's method, this is a lower order theme that is nested within a superordinate theme.

Subsumption. In Smith's interpretive phenomenological analysis, this occurs when an emergent theme itself is considered a superordinate theme as it assists in clustering a series of related themes.

Superordinate theme. A theme that represents higher order concepts that narratives share in Smith's interpretive phenomenological analysis.

Temporality. A fundamental lifeworld theme that refers to a person's subjective time and not clock time.

Textural-structural description. In Moustakas's modification, this description is constructed for each participant that includes the meanings and essences of their experience, incorporating the invariant constituents and themes.

Textural-structural synthesis. The final step in Moustakas's modification that involves an integration of the composite textural and composite structural descriptions to provide a synthesis of the meanings and essence of the experience.

Thoroughness. The evaluation criterion that examines whether the results convincingly addressed the research questions through completeness and saturation.

Triangulation. The process that involves using multiple sources of data and/or multiple methods of data collection.

Transferability. The degree to which qualitative results can be transferred to other groups or settings.

Trustworthiness. The amount of overall confidence readers of a qualitative study can have in the data collection and analysis based on Lincoln and Guba's criteria of credibility, dependability, confirmability, authenticity, and transferability.

Vividness. The evaluation criterion that examines if thick and faithful descriptions of the qualitative findings have been portrayed with clarity and artfulness.

Wholistic approach. van Manen's approach to uncovering themes when the researcher attends to the text as a whole.

Appendix A

First Study Activity for Students

Choose one of the phenomenological methodologies described in this text-book such as van Manen's or Giorgi's method. Using that person's name as one of your key terms, conduct a cross-disciplinary search for phenomenological studies on various databases such as Scopus, PubMED, CINAHL, psycINFO, ERIC, Social Work abstracts, socINDEX, and ABI/INFORM complete. Select one study and comment on its methodology using the following questions as a guide:

1. Did the study follow that specific phenomenological methodology? If not, which aspects of this methodology were not followed?

2. Was the research question congruent with that phenomenological approach?

3. Did the researchers describe the philosophical underpinning of their study? Was the type of phenomenology identified? Interpretive or descriptive phenomenology?

4. Was the sample size adequate and appropriate for that phenomenological methodology?

5. Was the data collection technique appropriate for that phenomenological methodology?

6. Was the data analysis approach appropriate for that phenomenological methodology? Did the researchers adequately describe the process used to analyze the data?

7. How well was that phenomenological research design described? Were any essential elements of that methodology missing?

8. Was there any evidence of method slurring?

9. If you were to conduct this phenomenological study using that methodology, are there any aspects of it you would change to strengthen its methodology?

Appendix B

Second Study Activity for Students

This second study activity is a discipline specific exercise. Using your discipline's primary database, such as ERIC for Education or psycINFO for Psychology, conduct a search for phenomenological studies published in the last 5 years. What type of phenomenology was published the most? Descriptive or interpretive? For descriptive phenomenological studies, what specific methodology was used most frequently in your discipline? Giorgi, Colaizzi, Dahlberg, van Kaam, Moustakas? What specific interpretive phenomenological methodology did researchers choose most often in your discipline? van Manen, Benner, Dahlberg, Smith?

Appendix C

Mothers' Experiences of Posttraumatic Growth Following Traumatic Childbirth:

A DESCRIPTIVE PHENOMENOLOGICAL STUDY PROPOSAL

Cheryl Tatano Beck, CNM, DNSc, FAAN
University of Connecticut

MOTHERS' EXPERIENCES OF POSTTRAUMATIC GROWTH FOLLOWING TRAUMATIC CHILDBIRTH

Posttraumatic growth has been reported among persons who have experienced a wide range of traumas. Examples of these trauma survivors include veterans (Tsai, El-Gabalawy, Sledge, Southwick, & Pietrzak, 2015), childhood cancer survivors (Duran, 2013), breast cancer survivors (Kolokotroni, Anagnostopoulos, & Tsikkinis, 2014), parents of children with cancer (Hullmann, Fedele, Moizon, Mayers, & Mullins, 2014), persons with chronic diseases of arthritis and inflammatory bowel disease (Purc-Stephenson, 2014), survivors of intimate partner violence (Valdez & Lilly, 2015), and women with infertility (Yu et al., 2014). The majority of research on posttraumatic growth in illness has focused on cancer as the leading illness studied. Only a handful of studies have been conducted on perinatal posttraumatic growth. None of these studies used a qualitative design to examine growth following birth trauma. Therefore, the purpose of this descriptive phenomenological study was to describe the essence of this growth experience in mothers who perceived their childbirth had been traumatic.

Posttraumatic growth is defined as the "positive psychological change experienced as a result of the struggle with highly challenging life circumstances" (Tedeschi & Calhoun, 2004, p. 1). In posttraumatic growth, a person's development in some areas surpasses what was present prior to the occurrence of the struggle with the crisis. Persons move beyond pretrauma levels in how they adapt (Tedeschi, Park, & Calhoun, 1998). A quality of transformation is involved in posttraumatic growth. This does not happen as a direct result of the trauma but instead as the result of the person's struggle in the aftermath of the trauma as they attempt to cope or survive. In this growth, the trauma does not disappear but still remains a distressing event. Posttraumatic growth can coexist with the distress of the trauma.

Posttraumatic growth involves three broad areas of growth: interpersonal, psychological, and life orientation changes (Tedeschi & Calhoun, 1995). Persons frequently reveal that their relationship with others is improved in some way, such as increased closeness. Second is a change in a person's self-perception, which may involve increased maturity or resilience. Third is a change in a person's philosophy of life, such as changes in life priorities. Tedeschi and Calhoun (1996) developed the Post-Traumatic Growth Inventory (PTGI), which measures perceived growth after trauma in five domains: new possibilities, relating to others, personal strength, spiritual change, and appreciation of life. A person can experience growth in some dimensions but not in all five domains. It must be noted that not all individuals who experience trauma develop posttraumatic growth.

Calhoun and Tedeschi (1998) used the metaphor of an earthquake to illustrate posttraumatic growth. When an individual experiences a traumatic event, the groundwork is laid for the potential of posttraumatic growth. Key to this development may be the traumatic event's ability to successfully "shake the foundations" of the person's assumptive world (p. 216). The trauma experience needs to be seismic, like in an earthquake, to achieve this severe shaking of a person's understanding of the world. As Calhoun and Tedeschi described, "a minimum threshold may need to be catastrophically crossed before events can have sufficient seismic power to produce the level of subjective disruption that is required for posttraumatic growth to be possible" (p. 216). These assumptions regarding the world that can be shaken include beliefs such as the meaning of life; why things happen to people; why persons think and act the way they do; relationships with other persons; one's abilities, strengths, weaknesses, and expectations for the future; spiritual or religious beliefs; and a person's worth or value as an individual (Cann et al., 2010). Cognitive rebuilding is necessary after a psychological crisis just as physical structures must be rebuilt after an earthquake.

PERINATAL POSTTRAUMATIC GROWTH

Posttraumatic growth in women after childbirth has been reported in three studies to date. Sawyer and Ayers (2009) were the first to conduct research on this topic. In their study, 219 women who had given birth within the previous 36 months (mean = 10.95 months) completed the PTGI (Tedeschi & Calhoun, 1996) and the Posttraumatic Stress Diagnostic Scale (PDS; Foa, Cashman, Jaycox, & Perry, 1997) via the Internet. Approximately 50% of this sample reported at least a moderate degree of positive change after childbirth. The domain of growth most frequently endorsed was appreciation of life, followed by personal strength, relating to others, new possibilities, and spiritual change. In the sample, 12.4% of the women met all the criteria necessary for PTSD related to childbirth. No significant relationship was found between PTSD symptoms and posttraumatic growth.

In Israel between 2008 and 2010, Taubman-Ben-Ari, Findler, and Sharon (2011) conducted a series of studies to assess the validity of the PTGI in measuring perceived growth related to the experience of motherhood. In Study 1,150 first-time mothers completed the PTGI and also answered the following open-ended statement: "Women who become mothers speak of various changes they experience. Please think about yourself and write down the changes that you have undergone following the transition to motherhood" (Taubman-Ben-Ari et al., 2011, pp. 607–608). Content analysis was used to analyze the open-ended statement and identify themes. The PTGI dimensions were compared to the themes. Four of the PTGI domains were reflected in the women's reports of the changes they had experienced in their lives following childbirth except for the domain of spirituality. These findings were confirmed in Study 2 with a sample of 157 first- and second-time mothers, mothers of singletons and twins, and mothers of preterm and full-term infants.

In 2012, Sawyer, Ayers, Young, Bradley, and Smith conducted a prospective study in the United Kingdom (UK) with 125 women who completed questionnaires during their third trimester and again 8 weeks postpartum. Women's posttraumatic stress symptoms during pregnancy were measured with the Impact of Event Scale-Revised (IES-R) (Weiss & Marmar, 1997). At 8 weeks postpartum, childbirth related PTSD symptoms were assessed using the PTSD Symptom Scale-Self Report (PSS-SR) (Foa, Riggs, Dancu, & Rothbaum, 1993). The PTGI (Tedeschi & Calhoun, 1996) measured growth after childbirth. In this sample, 23.2% of the mothers fulfilled the PTSD stressor criterion A regarding their childbirth. There were no significant differences in growth reported between mothers who did and did not fulfill stressor criterion A. Growth was significantly related to posttraumatic stress symptoms in pregnancy but not to posttraumatic stress symptoms related to birth. A multiple regression for predictors of total growth revealed that 32.3% of the variance in growth scores was explained by PTSD symptoms during pregnancy and cesarean birth (elective or emergency).

RESEARCH QUESTIONS

What is the essence of women's experiences of posttraumatic growth following birth trauma? What are the experiences of positive changes in mothers' beliefs or functioning that result from their struggles with traumatic childbirth?

RESEARCH DESIGN

Descriptive phenomenology is an inductive methodology that attempts to uncover and describe the essential structures of the lived experience of a phenomenon rather than transforming it into operationally defined behavior. One assumption of descriptive phenomenology is that for any human experience there are distinct essential structures that make up that phenomenon regardless of the particular person who experiences it. These essential structures are discovered by studying the particulars encountered in individual experiences. The essence of a phenomenon is grasped through the study of the particulars of experiences.

Husserl's (1970) philosophy of phenomenology underpins the descriptive phenomenological approach. The two steps of epoché and reduction are essential to Husserl's philosophy. Epoché means abstention, and reduction means to lead back. For Husserl, the epoché helps suspend our natural attitude of taken-for-granted beliefs of the phenomenon. He used the term "bracketing" for this first step, where one puts aside presuppositions that can stand in our way from being open to the phenomenon. Once bracketing is completed and we open ourselves to the world with our presuppositions, it leads to reduction, where one has transcendental access to the lifeworld and one can see what is unique in a phenomenon (Husserl, 1970).

Colaizzi's (1978) methodology called for researchers to uncover their presuppositions about the phenomenon being studied. He, however, stopped at having researchers completely bracket. Instead, Colaizzi (1978) instructed researchers to use their uncovered presuppositions to "interrogate" one's "beliefs, hypotheses, attitudes, and hunches" (p. 58).

SAMPLE

A sample of approximately 25 mothers will be projected to achieve the anticipated results of this qualitative study. Sample size in a qualitative study is typically small (Polit & Beck, 2017). Participants will be recruited until there is redundancy of the data with the participants' descriptions becoming repetitive with no new or different ideas. The meaningfulness and insights generated from qualitative data have more to do with the information richness of the participants' descriptions than with sample size.

There will be four criteria for inclusion in the study: (1) the participant is 18 years of age or older, (2) the participant perceives she had experienced a traumatic childbirth, (3) the woman can speak and read English, and (4) she can articulate her experience. Women of all ages and ethnic backgrounds are eligible to participate. Women will be recruited through a charitable trust in New Zealand, Trauma and Birth Stress (TABS), which was founded by five mothers who had experienced birth trauma. This self-help organization supports women who have experienced birth trauma and educates about birth trauma and the resulting PTSD. The co-investigator, Sue Watson, is the chairperson of TABS. Members of TABS will be informed of the study on their website (www.tabs .org.nz), where the recruitment notice will be posted. In addition, a recruitment notice will be placed in a parents' magazine, *Little Treasures*, in New Zealand to supplement the main recruitment site on TABS's website.

PROCEDURE

Prior to collecting and analyzing the data, the researcher will bracket her clinical experiences as a certified nurse-midwife caring for women who experienced traumatic births. She also will bracket the knowledge she has gained through her series of qualitative studies on birth trauma and its long-term negative consequences.

Recruitment will begin upon the University's Institutional Review Board approval. Women wanting information about the study will e-mail the researcher at her university address. Three documents will then be sent an attachment via e-mail to the potential participants: an information sheet, directions for the study, and a participant profile. Examples of demographic/obstetric variables asked for on the participant profile include age, marital status, educational level, number of children, and ethnicity. Mothers will be asked if they have been diagnosed with PTSD due to childbirth and if they are currently in therapy or counseling. In addition to completing a demographic and obstetric variables sheet, mothers will be asked to respond to the following statement: Please describe for us in as much detail as you can remember your experiences of any positive changes in your beliefs or life as a result of your traumatic childbirth. Potential participants will have the opportunity of e-mailing the researcher if they need any further clarification about the study before making their decision. Mothers sending their narratives to the researcher will imply informed consent. After reading a mother's description of her experiences of posttraumatic growth, the researcher may e-mail the participant if clarification of some part of her narrative is needed.

DATA ANALYSIS

Data from the study will be analyzed for common themes using Colaizzi's (1978) approach, which consists of the following steps:

- Read all the participants' descriptions of the phenomenon under study.

- Extract significant statements that pertain directing to the phenomenon.

- Formulate meanings for each significant statement.

- Categorize the formulated meanings into clusters of themes.

- Integrate the findings into an exhaustive description of the phenomenon being studied.

- Validate the exhaustive description by returning to some of the participants to ask them how it compares with their experiences.

- Incorporate any changes offered by the participants into the final description of the essence of the phenomenon.

METHODOLOGICAL RIGOR

Whittemore, Chase, and Mandle (2001) developed a synthesis of validity criteria gleaned from earlier published qualitative criteria. They organized the synthesis into primary criteria, which include credibility, authenticity, integrity, and criticality. Credibility refers to effort to establish confidence in the accuracy of the meanings of the findings. All interviews will be tape-recorded so that verbatim transcriptions are available to start data analysis. Insightful quotes of the mothers to give voice to each of the themes will be included. Authenticity is closely linked to credibility and focuses on the portrayal of the findings that reveal the experiences that are lived by the participants. Attention needs to be paid to subtle differences in the voices of mothers. This requires conscious attention to the influence of the researcher. The researcher will keep a reflexive journal to help her be aware of the influence of her perceptions, assumptions, etc., on the collection and analysis of the data. Criticality also involves the researcher critically appraising her exploration of negative instances, alternative hypotheses, and biases. Data will be analyzed with an eye to not avoiding any negative instances of the phenomenon. Peer debriefings with another qualitative researcher will periodically be held to guard against any distortions in the researcher's description of the phenomenon under study. Integrity focuses on the evidence that during each stage of the inquiry threats to researcher bias and her not paying attention to discrepant data are avoided. The researcher will be self-critical and demonstrate integrity at each phase of the study.

RISKS AND INCONVENIENCES

Even though women will be describing the positive changes in their life after their traumatic childbirth, remembering their birth trauma may cause an emotional response. If a mother should become anxious or upset, she will be told to take a break from writing her story. She may need to talk with her counselor/therapist, best friend, etc. The participant can also write in her story what it is that triggered her reaction now as she relives the event. The mother will be reminded that her participation in the study is voluntary and that she can withdraw at any time from the study without any consequences.

In the research report, quotes may be used, but any individually identifying information will be changed or deleted to protect confidentiality of the data collected. Participants will be warned, however, that since e-mail is not a secure transmission method, that their confidentiality cannot be guaranteed. For example, e-mail can be monitored by employers. Also, since e-mail is not encrypted, if the e-mail is somehow diverted or lost in transmission, the participant's story with her identification attached through her e-mail address can be exposed.

BENEFITS

While there will be no direct benefit for the women who participate in the study, the information they share will help health care professionals to provide better care for women who have experienced traumatic childbirth. Some mothers, however, have shared that they received a number of benefits as a result of participation in an interview about their traumatic births over the Internet via e-mail (Beck, 2005). There will be no costs to the participants, and no compensation will be provided.

REFERENCES

Beck, C. T. (2005). Benefits of participating in Internet interviews: Women helping women. *Qualitative Health Research, 15*, 411–422.

Cann, A., Calhoun, L. G., Tedeschi, R. G., Kilmer, R. P., Gil-Rivas, V., Vishnevsky, T., & Danhauer, S. C. (2010). The Core Beliefs Inventory: A brief measure of disruption in the assumptive world. *Anxiety, Stress, and Coping, 23,* 19–34.

Calhoun, L. G., & Tedeschi, R. G. (1998). Posttraumatic growth: Future directions. In R. G. Tedeschi, C. L. Park, & L. G. Calhoun (Eds.), *Posttraumatic growth: Positive change in the aftermath of crisis* (pp. 215–238). Mahwah, NJ: Lawrence Erlbaum Associates.

Colaizzi, P. (1978). Psychological research as the phenomenologist views it. In R. Valle & M. King (Eds.), *Existential phenomenological alternatives for psychology* (pp. 48–71). New York, NY: Oxford University Press.

Duran, B. (2013). Posttraumatic growth as experienced by childhood cancer survivors and their families: A narrative synthesis of qualitative and quantitative research. *Journal of Pediatric Oncology Nursing, 30,* 179–197.

Foa, E., Cashman, L., Jaycox, L., & Perry, K. (1997). The validation of a self-report measure of posttraumatic stress disorder: The Posttraumatic Stress Diagnostic Scale. *Psychological Assessment, 9,* 445–451.

Foa, E. B., Riggs, D. S., Dancu, C. V., & Rothbaum, B. O. (1993). Reliability and validity of a brief instrument for assessing post-traumatic stress disorder. *Journal of Traumatic Stress, 6,* 459–473.

Hullmann, S. E., Fedele, D. A., Moizon, E. S., Mayes, S., & Mullins, L. L. (2014). Posttraumatic growth and hope in parents of children with cancer. *Journal of Psychosocial Oncology, 32,* 696–707.

Husserl, E. (1970). *The crisis of European sciences and transcendental phenomenology: An introduction to phenomenology* (D. Carr, Trans.). Evanston, IL: Northwestern University Press.

Kolokotroni, P., Anagnostopoulos, F., & Tsikkinis, A. (2014). Psychosocial factors related to posttraumatic growth in breast cancer survivors: A review. *Women & Health, 54,* 569–592.

Polit, D. F., & Beck, C. T. (2017). *Nursing research: Generating and assessing evidence for nursing practice.* Philadelphia, PA: Wolters Kluwer.

Purc-Stephenson, R. J. (2014). The Posttraumatic Growth Inventory: Factor structure and invariance among persons with chronic diseases. *Rehabilitation Psychology, 59,* 10–18.

Sawyer, A., & Ayers, S. (2009). Post-traumatic growth in women after childbirth. *Psychology and Health, 24,* 457–471.

Sawyer, A., Ayers, S., Young, D., Bradley, R., & Smith, H. (2012). Posttraumatic growth after childbirth: A prospective study. *Psychology and Health, 27,* 362–377.

Taubman-Ben-Ari, O., Findler, L., & Sharon, N. (2011). Personal growth in mothers: Examination of the suitability of the Posttraumatic Growth Inventory as a measurement tool. *Women & Health, 51,* 604–622.

Tedeschi, R., & Calhoun, L. (1995). *Trauma and transformation: Growing in the aftermath of suffering.* Thousand Oaks, CA: SAGE.

Tedeschi, R., & Calhoun, L. (1996). The Posttraumatic Growth Inventory: Measuring the positive legacy of trauma. *Journal of Traumatic Stress, 9,* 455–472.

Tedeschi, R. G., & Calhoun, L. G. (2004). Posttraumatic growth: Conceptual foundations and empirical evidence. *Psychological Inquiry, 15,* 1–18.

Tedeschi, R., Park, C., & Calhoun, L. (1998). *Posttraumatic growth: Positive changes in the aftermath of a crisis*. Mahwah, NJ: Erlbaum.

Tsai, J., El-Gabalawy, R., Sledge, W. H., Southwick, S. M., & Pietrzak, R. H. (2015). Post-traumatic growth among veterans in USA: Results from the National Health and Resilience in Veterans Study. *Psychological Medicine, 45*, 165–179.

Valdez, C., & Lilly, M. M. (2015). Posttraumatic growth in survivors of intimate partner violence: An assumptive world process. *Journal of Interpersonal Violence, 30*, 215–231.

Weiss, D. S., & Marmar, C. R. (1997). The Impact of Event Scale—Revised. In J. P. Wilson & T. M. Keane (Eds.), *Assessing psychological trauma and PTSD: A handbook for practitioners* (pp. 399–411). New York, NY: Guilford.

Whittemore, R., Chase, S. K., & Mandle, C. L. (2001). Validity in qualitative research. *Qualitative Health Research, 11*, 522–537.

Yu, Y., Peng, L., Chen, L., Long, L., He, W., Li, M., & Wang, T. (2014). Resilience and social support promote posttraumatic growth of women with infertility: The mediating role of positive coping. *Psychiatry Research, 215*, 401–405.

Appendix D

The Impact of Traumatic Birth on Mothers Caring for Their Children:

AN INTERPRETIVE PHENOMENOLOGICAL STUDY PROPOSAL

Cheryl Tatano Beck, DNSc, CNM, FAAN
University of Connecticut

Up to 45% of new mothers have reported experiencing a traumatic birth (Alcorn, O'Donovan, Patrick, Creedy, & Devilly, 2010). Traumatic childbirth is an international public health problem, as reported, for example, in Japan (Takegata et al., 2017), Turkey (Gokce, Incl, Bektas, Yildiz, & Ayers, 2017), and the United Kingdom (Thomson & Downe, 2017). Yildiz, Ayers, and Phillips (2017) in their meta-analysis reported the mean prevalence of PTSD due to traumatic childbirth in community samples was 4.0% and 18.5% in high-risk groups. Traumatic childbirth has ever-widening ripple effects for mothers, such as impacting mothers' breastfeeding experiences, subsequent childbirths, and the anniversary of their traumatic births (Beck, 2015).

For a couple of decades now researchers have investigated the long-term effects that postpartum depression can have on mother-infant interactions and child development (Junge et al., 2017). Much less attention has been focused on the effects of posttraumatic stress on mother-infant attachment and child development. This study will help to fill this gap in the knowledge base. The purpose of this interpretive phenomenological study is to describe the impact of traumatic childbirth on mothers' experiences caring for their infants and older children.

LITERATURE REVIEW

A review of the literature revealed five qualitative studies that focused on the impact of traumatic childbirth on maternal-infant attachment and child development. Parfitt and Ayers (2009) examined the effects of posttraumatic stress disorder (PTSD) symptoms on mother-infant bonding. The sample of 126 mothers completed the Posttraumatic Stress Diagnostic Scale (Foa, Cashman, Jaycox, & Perry, 1997) and the Postpartum Bonding Questionnaire

(Brockington, Oates, George, & Turner, 2001) via an electronic survey. Seven women (5.6%) reported PTSD after childbirth. Women with PTSD symptoms reported a significantly poorer relationship with their infants. Structural equation modeling identified that PTSD symptoms had a direct effect on mother-baby bonding.

Enlow et al. (2011) found that maternal posttraumatic stress symptoms predicted infants' emotion regulation at 6 months of age in 52 mother-infant dyads. The sample primarily consisted of low income, ethnic/racial minority mothers and infants. Emotional regulation was assessed by the infant's ability to recover from distress during the Still-Face Paradigm (Haley & Stansbury, 2003) and mother's report of infant rate of recovery from distress/arousal in daily life. Maternal PTSD symptoms also predicted mothers' reports of infant externalizing, internalizing, and dysregulation symptoms at 13 months of age. Mothers also completed the PTSD Checklist-Civilian Version (Weathers, Huska, & Keane, 1991). In this sample, 27% of the women met the criteria for probable PTSD diagnosis.

Enlow et al. (2014) conducted a secondary analysis of their 2011 data set and this time focused on mother-infant attachment. Results revealed that elevated maternal PTSD symptoms at 6 months were significantly associated with increased risk for an insecure, disorganized mother-infant attachment relationship at 13 months postpartum.

Williams, Taylor, and Schwannauer (2016) enrolled 502 women in a web-based survey of mother-infant bonding, attachment experiences, and posttraumatic stress following childbirth. Women completed the Maternal Postnatal Attachment Scale (Condon & Corkindale, 1998), the Impact of Event Scale (Weiss & Marmar, 1997), and the Parental Bonding Instrument (Parker, Tupling, & Brown, 1979). By means of structural equation modeling, the researchers reported that posttraumatic stress was indirectly associated with mother-infant bonding. This relationship was mediated by depression.

The most recent study involved a population-based, 2-year follow-up study in Norway (Garthus-Niegel, Ayers, Martini, von Soest, & Ebserhard-Gran, 2017). Hospital birth records of 1,472 women were reviewed. At 8 weeks postpartum, women completed the Impact of Event Scale (Horowitz, Wilner, & Alvarez, 1979). When their children were 2 years old, mothers completed the Ages and Stages Questionnaire, which included four domains of child development. A significant longitudinal impact of postpartum PTSD symptoms on poor child social-emotional development was found 2 years later. This relationship remained significant even when adjusting for confounding variables of maternal depression, anxiety, and infant temperament.

RESEARCH QUESTION

What is the lived experience of the impact for mothers who have had a traumatic birth on caring for their children?

RESEARCH DESIGN

Interpretive phenomenology is an inductive methodology that attempts to uncover the essential structures of the lived experience of a phenomenon. Phenomenology is an approach to break through what we take for granted and allow one to get to the meaning structures of an experience. This basic methodology is based on reduction (Husserl, 1970) and consists of two steps that complement each other. First is bracketing, or epoché, where a person negatively suspends preconceptions about a phenomenon. The second step occurs when one positively returns to the phenomenon, allowing it to appear now that the natural attitude of taken-for-granted beliefs is suspended. Heidegger (1962) also stressed the significance of reduction but noted that reduction should not be viewed as a technique where one relies on a set of rules. One stays in the world of beings and does not suspend being in the world. For Heidegger, reduction is always incomplete. In hermeneutic reduction, one needs to be aware of his or her pre-understanding and theories about the phenomenon under study in order to achieve genuine openness in one's relationship with the phenomenon (van Manen, 2014). One can never totally forget our pre-understanding or vested interest. We need to continually practice critical self-awareness of perceptions that prevent us from being open to the phenomenon.

SAMPLE

Inclusion criteria for this sample will be that the woman (1) perceives her childbirth to have been traumatic, (2) is 18 years of age or older, and (3) is able to read and write English. Women of all ages and ethnic backgrounds are eligible to participate. Sample size in qualitative studies is typically small (Polit & Beck, 2017). Participants will be recruited until there is redundancy of the data, with the descriptions becoming repetitive with no new or different ideas.

Sample will be recruited from local obstetricians and nurse-midwifery practices. Recruitment notices will be posted in these practices' waiting rooms. The e-mail address and telephone numbers of the researcher will be included in the recruitment notice so that interested women can contact the researcher for more information about study participation.

RESEARCHER'S PERSPECTIVE

The researcher will practice reduction in order to be open to the phenomenon of traumatic birth and its impact on mothers' interactions with their children. Below is a summary of what the researcher will be aware of:

I have been researching traumatic births since 2001. I never had a traumatic birth myself, but as a nurse-midwife, I have cared for women who have. I have conducted a series of qualitative studies on birth trauma that include the following:

- Birth Trauma: In the Eye of the Beholder

- PTSD Following Childbirth: The Aftermath

- The Anniversary of Birth Trauma: Failure to Rescue

- The Impact of Traumatic Childbirth on Breastfeeding: A Tale of Two Pathways

- Subsequent Childbirth After a Previous Traumatic Birth

- Women's Experiences of EMDR Treatment for PTSD Due to Childbirth

From these qualitative studies, I have developed a mid-range theory of traumatic births that I entitled "The Ever-Widening Ripple Effect" (Beck, 2015).

PROCEDURE

After signing the informed consent, women will be asked to complete the Participant Profile, which asks for the following demographic and obstetric information: age, marital status, educational level, number of children, ethnicity, country of residence, type of birth, type of birth trauma, number of traumatic births they have had, do they have a history of prior trauma, whether or not they have been diagnosed with PTSD, and if they are currently in therapy or counseling. Next, women will be audiotaped as they are asked to respond to the following statement: "Please describe in as much detail as you can remember and wish to share how your traumatic birth has impacted your caring for and interactions with your infant and any other children you may have. Any specific examples you can share on your experiences will be extremely valuable in helping to educate clinicians so that they can provide better care to mothers who have experienced traumatic childbirth."

Participants who agree will be involved in a second interview to help the researcher interpret their transcripts from their first interviews. Women will be asked to bring a poem or a drawing or parts of a diary that can help explain their experiences of caring for their children after their traumatic birth.

DATA ANALYSIS

van Manen's (1997, 2014) approach to interpretive phenomenological research involves the following dynamic activities or processes:

1. Turning to a phenomenon that seriously interests us and commits us to the world

2. Investigating experience as we live it rather than as we conceptualize it

3. Reflecting on the essential themes that characterize the phenomenon

4. Describing the phenomenon through the art of writing and rewriting

In the first step, researchers are encouraged to focus on a human phenomenon that deeply interests them as the nature of lived experience. Lived experience is a person's immediate, prereflective self-awareness of life. Lived experience is both the starting point and end point of phenomenological research (van Manen, 1997). Also, step 1 includes formulating the research question.

Step 2 involves investigating experience as we live it. A researcher's personal experience is the starting point. Being aware of one's own experiences can provide the researcher with clues for orienting to the phenomenon under study. Next, data collection begins to obtain experiential descriptions from others. Participants can write their experiences, be interviewed, or be observed. The participants need to be guided to stay close to the experience as they lived it. Concrete examples are necessary and valuable. van Manen (1997, 2014) offers additional ways to develop a deeper understanding of the phenomenon under study, such as experiential descriptions in the literature, poetry, biographies, autobiographies, diaries, journals, and art.

Hermeneutic phenomenological reflection is the focus of step 3. Here the researcher tries to grasp the essential meaning of the phenomenon under study. The researcher reflects on lived experiences by analyzing the thematic aspects present in participants' experiences. Themes, according to van Manen (1997), are the structures of experience, the "knots in the webs of one's experiences" (p. 90). In other words, themes provide phenomenological power. van Manen described three approaches to uncover themes:

- Wholistic approach as one reads the text as a whole

- Selective, or highlighting, approach when one selects phrases or sentences that seem particularly revealing about the experience

- Detailed, or line-by-line approach where every single sentence is examined for what it reveals about the phenomenon

Interpretation through hermeneutic conversations with participants to reflect on ideal experiences once these have been gathered occurs in this step. A series of interviews can be arranged to allow a deeper reflection to provide more interpretive insight.

At this time, the researchers can also glean thematic descriptions from artistic sources. van Manen (1997) encouraged researchers to use literature, poetry, and biographies as sources for experiential material. He also suggested art as a source of lived experience such as paintings, sculpture, music, and cinematography. As themes emerged from this study on traumatic childbirth, this researcher will search these various sources to help bring these themes to their fullest light.

Step 4 entails hermeneutic phenomenological writing where the researcher writes up the findings from interpretive analysis of the participants' descriptions of their experiences of the phenomenon being studied.

PROTECTION OF HUMAN SUBJECTS

Once the research protocol is approved by the University of Connecticut's Institutional Review Board and the participant signs the informed consent, data collection will begin. The following procedures will be used to protect the confidentiality of the data. The researcher will keep all study records locked in a secure location. Participants will be labeled with a code. The code will be derived from a sequential 3-digit code that reflects how many people have enrolled in the study. The signed informed consents will be kept separately from the transcribed interviews. All electronic files (e.g., database, spreadsheet) will be password protected. Any computer hosting such files will also have password protection to prevent access by unauthorized users. Only the researcher will have access to the password.

Risk and Inconveniences:

We believe there are no known risks associated with this research study; however, participants will be told that if they become anxious describing the impact their traumatic births had on how they interacted with and cared for their children, they can stop participating in the study. They do not have to complete the study. One possible inconvenience to participants may be the time it takes to complete the interview.

Benefits:

Participants may not directly benefit from this research; however, we hope their participation in this survey will help health care professionals provide better care to mothers who have experienced a traumatic childbirth.

Economic Considerations:

There will be no costs to the participants, and they will not be paid to be in this study.

Trustworthiness:

Lincoln and Guba (1985) and Guba and Lincoln (1994) developed evaluative criteria for researchers to judge the quality of qualitative research. Trustworthiness includes the criteria of credibility, dependability, confirmability, transferability, and authenticity. Credibility focuses on the confidence one can have on the truth of the findings. Dependability looks at the stability of data over time and conditions. Confirmability addresses objectivity, meaning the congruence of two or more people about the data's meaning. Transferability refers to the degree to which results can have applicability in different settings and samples. Authenticity refers to the degree to which the researcher faithfully describes the range of realities.

Credibility will be addressed by producing interpretations from reflective writing, multiple interviews, observational notes, researcher's journal, and through interaction between and among participants and this researcher in multiple interviews. It will also be addressed by explicating the researcher's understandings, beliefs, biases, assumptions, presuppositions, and theories.

"We try to come to terms with our assumptions not in order to forget them again, but rather to hold them deliberatively at bay and even to turn this knowledge against itself, as it were, thereby exposing its shallow or concealing character" (van Manen, 1997, p. 47).

Transferability will be established by producing thick descriptions of the impact of traumatic childbirth on mothers' experiences interacting with their children. Dependability deals with the reliability or consistency of the study. Lincoln and Guba (1985) argued that since there can be no validity without reliability, there can be no credibility without dependability. Dependability will be established by clearly documenting every decision and interpretation strategy throughout the research process. Confirmability will be achieved by analyzing the data together with the participants. Multiple interviews will allow the researcher and the participant a second chance to make sure that the data were interpreted correctly or understanding occurred. Authenticity will be addressed by face-to-face interviews with participants. Quotes from mothers will be included in the description of the themes to bring to life the voices of the women.

REFERENCES

Alcorn, K. L., O'Donovan, A., Patrick. J. C., Creedy, D., & Devilly, G. J. (2010). A prospective longitudinal study of the prevalence of posttraumatic stress disorder resulting from childbirth events. *Psychological Medicine, 40,* 1849–1859.

Beck, C. T. (2015). Middle range theory of traumatic childbirth: The ever-widening ripple effect. *Global Qualitative Nursing Research*, 1–13. doi: 10.1177/23 33393615575313

Brockington, I., Oates, J., George, S., & Turner, D. (2001). A screening questionnaire for mother-infant bonding disorders. *Archives of Women's Mental Health*, 3, 133–140.

Condon, J. T., & Corkindale, C. J. (1998). The assessment of parent-to-infant attachment: Development of a self-report questionnaire. *Journal of Reproductive and Infant Psychology, 16*, 57–76.

Enlow, M. B., Egeland, B., Carlson, E., Blood, E., & Wright, R. J. (2014). Mother-infant attachment and the intergenerational transmission of posttraumatic stress disorder. *Developmental Psychopathology, 26*, 41–65.

Enlow, M. B., Kitts, R. L., Blood, E., Bizarro, A., Hofmeister, M., & Wright, R. J. (2011). Maternal posttraumatic stress symptoms and infant emotional reactivity and emotion regulation. *Infant and Behavioral Development, 34*, 487–503.

Foa, E. B., Cashman, L., Jaycox, L., & Perry, K. (1997). The validation of a self-report measure of posttraumatic stress disorder: The Posttraumatic Diagnostic Scale. *Psychological Assessment, 9*, 445–451.

Garthus-Niegel, S., Ayers, S., Martini, J., von Soest, T., & Eberhard-Gran, M. (2017). The impact of postpartum posttraumatic stress disorder symptoms on child development: A population-based, 2-year follow-up study. *Psychological Medicine, 47*, 161–170.

Gokce, I. G., Incl, F., Bektas, M., Yildiz. P. D., & Ayers, S. (2017). Risk factors associated with post-traumatic stress symptoms following childbirth in Turkey. *Midwifery, 41*, 96–103.

Guba, E. G., & Lincoln, Y. S. (1994). Competing paradigms in qualitative research. In N. Denzin & Y. Lincoln (Eds.), *Handbook of qualitative research* (pp. 105–117). Thousand Oaks, CA: SAGE.

Haley, D. W., & Stansbury, K. (2003). Infant stress and parent responsiveness: Regulation of physiology and behavior during still-face and reunion. *Child Development, 74*, 1534–1546.

Heidegger, M. (1962). *Being and time.* New York, NY: Harper and Row.

Horowitz, M., Wilner, N., & Alvarez, W. (1979). Impact of Event Scale: A measure of subjective stress. *Psychosomatic Medicine, 41*, 209–218.

Husserl, E. (1970). *The crisis of European sciences and transcendental phenomenology* (D. Carr, Trans.). Evanston, IL: Northwestern University Press.

Junge, C., Garthus-Niegel, S., Slinning, K., Polte, C., Simonsen, T. B., & Eberhard-Gran, M. (2017). The impact of perinatal depression on children's social-emotional development: A longitudinal study. *Maternal Child Health Journal, 21,* 607–615.

Lincoln, Y. S., & Guba, E. G. (1985). *Naturalistic inquiry.* Newbury Park, CA: SAGE.

Parfitt, Y., & Ayers, S. (2009). The effect of post-natal symptoms of post-traumatic stress and depression on the couples' relationship and parent-baby bond. *Journal of Reproductive and Infant Psychology, 27,* 127–142.

Parker, G., Tuping, H., & Brown, L. B. (1979). A parental bonding instrument. *British Journal of Medical Psychology, 52,* 1–10.

Polit, D. F., & Beck, C. T. (2017). *Nursing research: Generating and assessing evidence for nursing practice.* Philadelphia, PA: Wolters Kluwer.

Takegata, M., Haruna, M., Matsuzaki, M., Shiraishi, M., Okano, T., & Severinsson, E. (2017). Aetiological relationships between factors associated with postnatal traumatic symptoms among Japanese primiparas and multiparas: A longitudinal study. *Midwifery, 44,* 14–23.

Thomson, G., & Downe, S. (2017). Emotions and support needs following a distressing birth: Scoping study with pregnant multigravida women in North-West England. *Midwifery, 40,* 32–39.

Van Manen, M. (1997*). Researching lived experience: Human science for an active sensitive pedagogy.* Ontario, Canada: The State University of New York.

Van Manen, M. (2014). *Phenomenology of practice.* Walnut Creek, CA: Left Coast Press.

Weathers, F. W., Huska, J. A., & Keane, T. M. (1991). The PTSD Checklist-Civilian Version (PCL-C). Available from F. W. Weathers, National Center for PTSD, Boston Veterans Affairs Medical Center, 150 S. Huntington Avenue, Boston, MA 02130.

Weiss, D. S., & Marmar, C. R. (1997). The Impact of Event Scale—Revised. In J. P. Wilson & T. M. Keane (Eds.), *Assessing psychological trauma and PTSD* (pp. 399–411). New York, NY: Guilford Press.

Williams, C., Taylor, E. P., & Schwannauer, M. (2016). A web-based survey of mother-infant bond, attachment experiences, and metacognition in posttraumatic stress following childbirth. *Infant Mental Health Journal, 37,* 259–273.

Yildiz, P. D., Ayers, S., & Phillips, L. (2017). The prevalence of posttraumatic stress disorder in pregnancy and after birth: A systematic review and meta-analysis. *Journal of Affective Disorders, 208,* 634–645.

Index

Negative case analysis, 119 (table), 120
Noronha, E., 78–79
Nutting, R., 101
Nyström, M., 57–65, 103,
110–112 (table), 150. *See also*
Reflective lifeworld methodology

Objectivity, 1, 118
Observation, 76, 90, 120
Ontology, 13
Open listening, 84–85
Openness, 57, 58, 59, 103–104, 105.
See also Bridling; Reduction
Osborn, M., 96

Page limitations, 133
Paradigm cases, 85–86
Parenthesizing, 12. *See also* Bracketing/
epoché; Reduction
Parfitt, Y., 187
Participant observation, 90
Participants
in Colaizzi's approach, 36
confidentiality of, 133, 183, 192
consent and, 162, 192
as coresearchers, 21
developing research program and,
141–142
in Giorgi's approach, 36
insight into experience of, 1–2.
See also Lived experience
number of. *See* Sample
protection of, 192
in research proposal, 192
returning to, 23, 65, 68, 106, 120.
See also Member checking
risks and inconveniences to,
182–183, 192
as subjects, 44
in van Kaam's approach, 44
See also Sample
Peer review/debriefing, 119 (table),
120
Perception, 14
Petri, S., 62, 62 (table)
Phenomenology
defined, 11
described, 73
evaluating. *See* Evaluating research

as science of examples, 73
use of, 1–2
Phenomenology, descriptive, 2. *See also*
Methodologies, descriptive
Phenomenology, interpretive/
hermeneutic, 2. *See also*
Methodologies, interpretive/
hermeneutic
Phenomenology of Perception
(Merleau-Ponty), 14
Phillips, L., 187
Philosophy of phenomenology, 2
Gadamer, 15, 57, 59, 130
Heidegger, 13–14, 83, 149, 150, 189
Husserl, 11–13, 14, 31, 32, 34, 57,
150, 180
Merleau-Ponty, 14–15, 20, 57, 150
Picton, C., 50
Polit, D. F., 120
Postpartum depression, 23–25
Posttraumatic stress disorder (PTSD),
research program on, 141–145
Preconceptions, 84. *See also* Bracketing/
epoché; Reduction
Presentation
of descriptive phenomenology
studies, 60
of IPA, 97
qualitative reporting checklists,
137–138
See also Writing, phenomenological
Presuppositions, 12, 19–20. *See also*
Bracketing/epoché; Natural
attitude; Reduction
Pre-understanding, 105. *See also*
Bracketing/epoché; Reduction
Prior knowledge. *See* Bracketing/epoché;
Natural attitude; Reduction
Procedure, in research proposal,
181, 190
Prose of the World (Merleau-Ponty), 15
PTSD (posttraumatic stress disorder),
research program on, 141–145
Pulvirenti, M., 77–78
Qualitative research
evaluating. *See* Evaluating research
phenomenology and, 1
vs. quantitative research, 117–118
trustworthiness in, 117–127

in van Manen's approach, 75
See also Participants
Sandelowski, M., 131
Sanders, S., 78
Sawyer, A., 178, 179
Schwannauer, M., 188
Science, loss of meaning for life, 11
Second person perspective, 149
Shankar, J., 27
Sharon, N., 179
Sidenius, U., 63
Significant statements, examples of,
    152–156 (table), 156, 157 (table)
Situation, 87
Sivberg, B., 36–37
Smith, H., 179
Smith, J. A., 93–101, 113, 124, 150.
    See also Interpretive
    phenomenological analysis (IPA)
Software, qualitative, 163
Spatiality, 77, 78, 80
Spiral, 59, 105, 113. *See also*
    Hermeneutical rule/circle/spiral
Standards for Reporting Qualitative
    Research (SRQR), 137–138
Stensland, M., 78
Stretton-Smith, P. A., 99, 100, 101 (figure)
Structure, 32. *See also* Essence
Studies, phenomenological
    developing research program,
        141–145
    lack of methodological rigor, 2–3
    See also Evaluating research;
        Methodologies; Quality of
        research; Research program;
        Research proposal; Rigor
Study activities, 7, 175
    evaluating phenomenological study, 127
    evaluating studies, 173
    for writing, 138–139
Subjects, 44. *See also* Participants
Sullivan, N. B., 52, 53 (table), 54
Sumskis, S., 49
Svanström, R., 108

Tangvald-Petersen, O., 37
Taubman-Ben-Ari, O., 179

Taylor, E. P., 188
Teaching phenomenology, 147–164
    phenomenology tips, 160–163
    strategies for, 147–160
    teaching Colaizzi's approach,
        150–151, 152–156 (table),
        156, 158
Tedeschi, R. G., 137, 178
Temporality, 77, 78, 80, 87, 113
Terminology, 118
Text, dialoguing with, 104–105
Textorium, 129
Thematic analysis, 86
Themes
    in Colaizzi's methodology, 23
    essential, 77
    in Smith's methodology, 95–96
    uncovering, 77, 79
    in van Manen, 77
Theoretical coalescence, 143
Thorne, S., 131, 132 (table), 133
Titles, 133–134
Tolotti, A., 90
Transcriptionists, 162–163
Transferability, 118,
    121–122 (table), 193
Transformation of participant's data,
    32, 34
Transformed meaning, 34–35, 35 (table)
Traumatic childbirth. *See* Birth trauma
Triangulation, 119 (table), 120
Trustworthiness, 117–127
    criteria for, 118, 121–122 (table)
    vs. reliability and validity, 117–120
    in research proposal, 193
Truth and Method (Gadamer), 15
Turok, D. K., 52

Understanding
    Gadamer on, 15
    tracking steps in, 84
Ungar, M., 99
Usman, D. J., 89
Utrecht School of phenomenology, 73

Validation, 23, 65, 87. *See also* Member
    checking; Participants, returning to

Ingram Content Group UK Ltd.
Milton Keynes UK
UKHW021944090523
421477UK00014B/314

9 781544 319551